NO MORE BACK PAIN

NO MORE BACK PAIN

*A New and Proven Program to
Free Yourself from Back Pain for Life*

Alfred O. Bonati, M.D.
Shirley Linde, Ph.D.

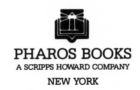

PHAROS BOOKS
A SCRIPPS HOWARD COMPANY
NEW YORK

As in any medical program, this plan should be followed under the guidance and supervision of a physician.

Interior design: Joan Greenfield

First published in 1991.

Library of Congress Cataloging-in-Publication Data:
Bonati, Alfred O.
No more back pain : a proven program to free yourself from back pain for life / Alfred O. Bonati and Shirley Linde.
p.   cm.
Includes index.
ISBN 0-88687-525-0 : $18.95
1. Backache—Popular works. I. Linde, Shirley Motter.
II. Title.
RD771.B217B66   1991
617.5'64—dc20   91-17072   CIP

Printed in the United States of America

Pharos Books
A Scripps Howard Company
200 Park Avenue
New York, N.Y. 10166

10 9 8 7 6 5 4 3 2 1

Contents

CHAPTER ONE

Why You Should Be Concerned About Your Back

On Monday morning Peter was getting ready for work when he sneezed, hard. The next thing he knew he was lying on the floor in excruciating pain, unable to move.

"My back's out," he thought, although he was only guessing because he had never had any back trouble in his life.

Helen's back trouble came on more slowly. At first she developed back pain after an afternoon weeding the garden; then that autumn the pain was even worse after raking leaves. Before she knew it, her back started hurting after every little bit of exertion. Today she is in pain constantly.

It could happen to almost anyone. It may have already happened to you.

Most of us take our backs for granted. We assume that they will continue to function without trouble throughout life. But the chances are good that most of us, even if we have a back that seems normal, either have already had episodes of back pain or have a good chance of suffering back pain and disability in the future.

It could happen gradually with everyday strains, tension, and lack of exercise gradually causing nagging pains. Or it may happen suddenly with no warning. You could be shoveling snow, or bending over to raise a stuck window, or simply reaching down to pick something up off the floor, when a stab of pain rips through your back, and you may not be able to straighten up.

The Facts on Backs

The most recent statistics show that almost everyone has a back problem at one time or another. In fact, one government survey shows that back problems are now reported to be the number one complaint of patients going to the doctor, even more than sore throats, colds, and stomachaches.

And a bad back is the second most frequent cause of absenteeism from work. (Colds and flu are number one.)

Frighteningly, the problem is getting worse—throughout the medical profession we are finding a shocking increase in both the frequency and severity of back problems. More and more people are being affected every year, so that today, back problems have reached epidemic proportions, touching every segment of the population. In fact, one research report indicated that, in the area studied, low back disability was increasing 14 times faster than was the growth in population. It is now estimated that four out of every five people in the United States can expect to experience back trouble at some time in their lives!

Here are even more shocking statistics on back pain.

It is estimated that some 80 million people in the United States suffer from some type of back pain. Of these, health insurance companies report that about 28 million victims hobble their way into doctors' offices or clinics like ours for treatment each year, and on any given day, 6.5 million people are in bed because of back pain. Many others have pain and stiffness and lack of mobility, but have not yet gone to seek professional help.

At some back pain clinics there is a five- to six-month waiting list to get an appointment because so many people need help.

Some $20 *billion*, some say $50 billion, is reportedly spent annually on back care and back products. The expenses to an individual patient can be truly astronomical. One woman we talked to reported expenses of $160,000 over eight years. One man told us he spent $450,000 out of his and his insurance company's pocket. The emotional cost of pain to individuals and families in terms of unhappiness and crippled lives is even higher.

The cost to society is high in lost wages and productivity and in compensation payments. An estimated 2 million Americans with back problems cannot hold jobs, and 5 million are partially disabled. Back pain accounts for 93 million days of work lost and more than $10 billion in Worker's Compensation claims. In some states 75 percent of all compensation payments go to back patients. In fact, bad backs are the number one claim filed on disability insurance policies.

A Pain in the Back Is Not Normal

Back pain has become so common that many people simple live with their pain and misery, accepting it stoically as a natural part of their lives.

But most back pain that people suffer is unnecessary and can be prevented or treated. People do not need to have back pain. Things can be done. The spine is not just an anatomical hat rack on which you hang your body's muscles and organs; it can be strengthened and made more flexible with conditioning. There are techniques to tone the muscles, improve posture, stretch ligaments, increase flexibility, reduce pain, and increase function.

Many of these techniques have evolved in only the last few years, changing tremendously doctors' knowledge about back pain and how to treat it. But most of this new knowledge has not yet reached the public. That is why we have written this book. The book, and the healing program described in it include these new concepts and latest treatments.

The patients described have been treated at the Gulf Coast Orthopedic Center (GCOC) Institute for Special Surgery in Hudson, Florida. The Institute, just north of Tampa and St. Petersburg, was founded in 1981 for special surgery of joint diseases. Now patients come to the Institute from around the world for relief of pain of their shoulders, knees, necks, hips, and especially their backs. Health practitioners come also—to study the innovative techniques developed and used at the Institute.

The techniques have been dramatically effective—patients come in on crutches or on stretchers and walk out without pain under their own power.

We have put these techniques—those developed at the Institute and those developed elsewhere—into a complete healing program, most of which you can do at home yourself.

The program has been used at the GCOC Institute in one phase or another in more than 5,000 back patients.

The results show that back sufferers not only can be helped, but in an amazing number of cases, they can be helped without drugs or surgery. Even persons who are about to undergo surgery can often have their backs strengthened considerably by doing exercises before surgery. After surgery, patients can do the exercises to help restore their back strength and help prevent further injury. Sometimes the preoperative exercises make it possible to even avoid surgery altogether. If surgery is necessary, the new techniques of surgery can make it possible for the patient to be up and walking the next day.

One new technique developed at the GCOC Institute is arthroscopy for the back. Like arthroscopy of the knee, a tiny incision allows the surgeon to see inside the joints while working from the outside and viewing the work on a television monitor. This new technique plus the exercise program and physical therapy developed there, as described in this book, have relieved pain in 91 percent of the patients treated.

Bill was a typical example. He came into the clinic with terrible pain—advanced degenerative disc disease. He was only 44 years old, but had already had a spinal surgery. He had constant back pain, plus pain that radiated down into his right leg. It was even worse when he tried to sit, twist, or stand. The pain kept him awake most nights, and he could walk no more than three blocks before the pain became so excruciating that he had to stop even that. Surgery was done at the GCOC Institute with the new techniques, Bill did the exercises described in our book, and other forms of physical therapy were administered. The result: He became totally free of pain, has returned to work, and is doing well.

Often our patients say that they found relief for their back pain for the first time. Nothing before had ever worked.

Whether you have a bad back and want to make it stronger, have a good back and want to make it even better, or want to prevent future problems, we believe that this book will help you.

You May Be Now Doing All the Wrong Things

Often back troubles occur because people unknowingly do the wrong things to their backs. The wrong kind of exercises, even common ones, can aggravate a back problem. Even simple exercises like bending down and touching your toes can cause back damage. In fact, doctors report that many patients come to them with problems caused by improper exercises that have however been recommended in exercise programs, and they warn that even some of the exercises taught to schoolchildren are dangerous. The exercises that are taught in most fitness programs are exercises developed for the general population, not for people with bad backs.

You may be exercising, but you may be doing sit-ups or toe touches when you should not be. You may be running up and down steep hills instead of on flat ground or swimming the breaststroke instead of the crawl.

The concept of exercises for the back have changed over recent years. In *No More Back Pain* we bring you the most up-to-date information in a step-by-step healing program, including exercises designed specifically for strengthening the back. They are effective and safe.

How you drive your car, the chairs you sit on, the mattresses you choose (even expensive ones), how you do things at home and at work—all can aggravate a back problem. You may even be getting out of bed improperly.

If you already have back trouble, even mild trouble, then naturally if you keep doing the wrong things, you will have worse trouble in the future. Today's twinge can be tomorrow's excruciating pain that could cripple your back and your life. That first back pain is your back's signal for help, and unless you do something now, you may have a bigger problem in the future.

You Can Have a Strong Back

The program in this book will give you specific guidelines that you can follow to help prevent the wrong—the harmful— situations. It will tell you right things to do, the simple steps to take to improve your back now, and the steps needed to prevent trouble in the future. It will teach you how to bend, sit, lift, run, reach a high shelf, and exit a car without insulting your back.

The program gives you conditioning exercises and other advice gathered from back experts around the world. By learning the techniques and following the program, you can strengthen key muscles and stretch tight areas, so that you can begin to restore your back to normal function and eliminate pain for good.

The steps are easy to follow and take only a few minutes a day—mostly flat on your back. More important, nothing in the program is damaging or pain producing. And the program works. Even if your back now hurts you every day, the program can give you a chance to once more have a good back so you can live with more vigor, walk without pain, and feel and look better again.

CHAPTER TWO

Home Back Tests You Can Do Right Now

Back problems can sneak up on you, so it can pay to find out now whether your back is starting to become weak or to have other problems. Then you can get started on strengthening your back before serious trouble starts.

Back tests done at home do not take the place of a regular physical checkup, but they are a safe, acceptable way to get started on finding abnormalities or weaknesses that could mean trouble in you or a member of your family. If you find any symptoms or signs of a problem, or anything that is question-able, see your doctor and tell him or her what you found.

We want you to do the tests slowly and smoothly, in comfortable clothes and with your shoes off. Do *not* warm up your muscles by exercising or bathing before you take the tests.

But, first, you should know some facts about your back.

The Anatomy of the Back

The back is an engineering marvel. With its 33 vertebrae, it supports most of the body's weight and allows us to stand up, bend, twist, and swivel. It protects 31 pairs of nerves with branches going to and from the brain and to all parts of the body, carrying every sensation for pain, touch, heat, and cold and every signal for muscle action that your body knows about. It has three layers of sheathing and a cushiony fluid bath to protect the nerves.

The spine has an S-shape—a brilliant design that acts as its own shock absorber—and for additional shock absorption, it has discs between each vertebra, something like jelly-filled doughnuts, with a tough outer cartilage cover and a gel-like interior that cushions every step you take. There are more than 400 intricately connected muscles and 1,000 ligaments supporting the system, giving you shape, support, and most of your ability to move.

Starting from the top and working down, the lineup of your spine is as follows:

The Cervical Spine   This is the neck region, with seven vertebrae. The top one, called the atlas, supports and balances your head on the top of your spine. The flexibility of the cervical vertebrae makes it possible for you to move your head through a wide range of positions. The last cervical vertebra, C7, is where you feel the big bump at the back of your neck between your shoulders.

The Thoracic or Dorsal Spine   Going from the bottom of your neck to your waist, the thoracic (or dorsal) spine consists of 12 vertebrae. Their main function is to connect to and support the ribs.

The Lumbar Spine   The lower back region. It has five large vertebrae that support most of the body weight and work like a pivot between the upper and lower parts of the body. This five-piece pivot absorbs most of the stress and strain of the back and is the area that most frequently gives trouble.

The Sacrum The five vertebrae of the sacrum are actually fused into one solid triangular structure that is connected to the two big bones of the pelvis called the *ilia*, making up the *sacroiliac joint*. It provides a place for your hip bones to attach your legs to your body. Although the sacroiliac joint has often

THE ANATOMY OF THE SPINE

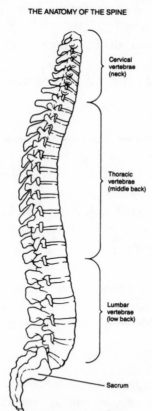

Cervical vertebrae (neck)

Thoracic vertebrae (middle back)

Lumbar vertebrae (low back)

Sacrum

Coccyx

been blamed for backache, it seldom causes trouble except in some cases of arthritis, or if injured.

The Coccyx This is your tailbone, consisting of four vertebrae fused together. It does little but give some connection to the small rectal muscles that control bowel movements. The tailbone is actually the remnant of what was once a tail in early evolution.

Ligaments and Tendons

Ligaments (they connect bones to bones) join together the little projections of the vertebrae to provide support as you move forward and bend backward and to prevent you from tipping over sideways when you stand up.

Tendons connect muscles to bones and make it possible for the muscles to move the bones.

Muscles That Affect Your Back

A muscle does its work by contracting and getting shorter. It relaxes and gets longer when resting. The rather neat design scheme is that muscles always work in pairs: if a muscle contracts to bend your back to the right, then the opposite muscle has to be relaxed to let it go. The teamwork happens automatically. When the nerve impulse sends the signal to make one muscle contract, it also sends an inhibitory impulse to the opposing muscle so it will not contract.

It is when your muscles are strained with too hard a pull or too long a constant contraction that you can have pain.

The four major muscle groups of the back are the following:

- *The spine extensors.* These muscles are in layers and are attached to the spine, pelvis, and ribs.
- *The lateral muscles.* These are located along each side of the spine. The two most important are the *quadratus lumborum*, which balances the sideways motions of the spine, and the

psoas major, which flexes the trunk and continues down to the hip joint to rotate the hips.

- *Abdominal muscles.* These sheets of muscle support the abdomen and help to support and balance the movements of the back.
- *Hip muscles.* These are connected to the pelvis and the spine. They help you to flex your hips by raising your thighs, and help you to balance on your two legs, walk, climb, and run.

You will find out more about where some of these bones and muscles are as you do the tests in this chapter.

The Many Causes of Back Pain

The tests you will do in this chapter may enable you to find the problems that could be causing your back pain, but you need to be aware that there are many possible causes of back pain and many of these conditions can only be diagnosed and treated by a physician.

Most commonly, a case of back pain, especially pain in the lower back, comes from an injured muscle or ligament (perhaps from a sudden twist or a fall). Also common is pain caused by injury to a vertebra or degeneration of a spinal disc, the jellylike cushion between the vertebrae. There may be minor damage; the disc may be bulging, causing pain from the stretching. Or the outer ring of the disc (the *annulus*) may be torn and the softer center pushed partly out, called a ruptured disc. If there is pressure on a spinal nerve, pain may occur in the hip, leg, or foot—an important clinical sign used by the physician to determine which nerve is involved in your problem.

But there can be many other causes, even seemingly unrelated things, things you might never think of, such as an infection, an ulcer, prostate problems, emotional tension, an aneurysm, or cancer. If you are a cigarette smoker, constant coughing could be putting a strain on your spine.

It could be something simple—you may have been spading the garden when you were out of shape. Or it could be something complicated and less obvious—such as a kidney disorder or referred pain from some internal organ. And to make it even more complicated, there may not be a single cause, but several causes involved, one aggravating the other. In children, back pain often is associated with development of a crooked spine (*scoliosis*) or a tumor of the spine and needs immediate attention.

Some causes are rare, but it is important to consider all the possibilities, because only by knowing the cause can your doctor recommend the right treatment. Looking over the list, you'll see why finding the cause of a person's back pain is not simple.

Here are some of the causes of back pain:

Injury caused by a blow to a vertebra

Fall from a height, causing sudden compression of the vertebra and discs

Strain from lifting an awkward or heavy object

Muscle strain during pregnancy

Muscle spasm

Not enough exercise

Improper exercise

Sleeping on a poor mattress

Poor posture when standing, sitting, or walking

Flabby abdominal muscles

Overweight

Foot disorder, such as fallen arches

Improper shoes

Imbalance of muscles of the back and legs

One leg shorter than the other
Vitamin deficiencies
Emotional tension
Arthritis
Osteoporosis
Bulging or ruptured disc
Fracture of the vertebra
Narrowing of the spinal canal opening
Formation of a spur on a vertebra
Infection of the spine or spinal fluid
Kidney trouble
Disorder of the uterus
Prostate trouble
Tumor (benign or cancerous)
Metabolic disease
Hormone change of menopause
Referred pain from pneumonia
Referred pain from an ulcer
Cancer that has spread from other sites, especially from the lung
Pancreatic disease
Circulatory disorder, including arteriosclerosis
Aneurysm (dangerous ballooning and weakening of an artery)
Liver disorder
Gallbladder disease
Disease of the reproductive organs
Nerve disorder
Bone disease

Tests for Adults

First, Check for More Serious Trouble Signs

To check out someone's back, run your fingers carefully down his or her spine. Feel for any especially deep indentations or blank spaces between the vertebrae and for any small masses or strange extra lumps.

Check both sides of the spinal column for areas of increased oil or sweat or groups of hairs in patches or in a tuft like a small brush. These often indicate congenital abnormalities in the spine underneath.

Press all along the spine, along the pelvic bones, and over the lower back on each side to see if there is any tenderness.

If the person has any of these signs, you should contact a physician, since they could indicate something as serious as *spina bifida*, a condition in which the spine is incompletely formed, or a tumor.

Then, Check for Swayback (Lordosis)

Stand sideways and observe your posture in a full-length mirror, or have the person you are checking stand sideways in front of you.

Compare the curve in your back with the posture shown in the accompanying figure.

It is normal for the back to have a slight curve, but too much of a curving arch is called *lordosis* (or swayback) and puts a strain on the back that can lead to trouble.

A Quiz for Muscle Imbalance

Many people have muscle imbalance—the muscles are shorter or tighter on one side of the body, throwing the body a tiny bit off balance. Or the body may be off balance due to one leg being slightly shorter than the other. Muscle imbalance or

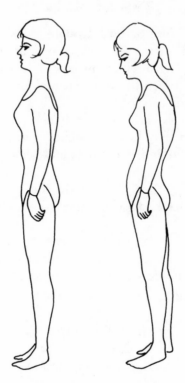

NORMAL VERSUS SWAYBACK

short-leg syndrome often can lead to pains in the back or in the legs, knees, thighs, or neck.

Look through the following checklist of clues that could mean you have an imbalance.

- Do you sometimes need to have slacks altered because one pants leg is a little too long, or does the hem of a new dress or skirt frequently need to be evened?

16

- Does your slip or T-shirt tend to slip off one shoulder more than the other because one shoulder tends to be higher than the other?
- Do your feet turn in or out, or do you often stumble or fall over your own feet? Do you sprain your ankles often?
- Do you have bunions, painful heel spurs, or thick calluses where your shoes rub your feet? Do the heels wear down more quickly on one side of your shoes than the other?
- Do you get neck, shoulder, or backaches during long car rides?
- Do you slouch when you sit or stand?

If you find that you have signs of crooked spine, swayback, or muscle imbalance, call them to the attention of your physician at your next examination. They may be so slight that nothing needs to be done, but they may be serious enough to require attention.

Checking for Flexibility
To check for flexibility, stand straight, then bend at the waist to the right and to the left, then again standing up straight, twist to the right and to the left. Is there freedom of motion, or is there stiffness and limited motion, or pain?

Sit on the floor, upright and straight (not leaning backward) and with the legs fully extended straight ahead. You should be able to keep the legs fully extended and flat to the floor without pain or difficulty and without falling backward.

Tests for Muscle Strength
(If you have back trouble, or any serious health problems, or are pregnant, check with your physician before taking these tests. If you feel pain at any time while taking the tests, stop doing them and do not take further tests or do back exercises without first checking with your doctor.)

17

1. Lie flat on your back on the floor, hands clasped behind your neck, legs straight and touching. Keep your knees straight and lift your feet 10 inches above the floor.
2. Still flat on the floor, with hands clasped behind your neck, have someone hold down your legs by grasping the ankles, or hook your ankles under a heavy chair that won't topple. Roll up into a sitting position. Make sure you roll gently; don't lurch as you might in a regular sit-up.
3. Still on the floor, with hands behind your neck, bend your knees with your heels close to your buttocks. Again, have someone hold your ankles down or hook them under something sturdy. Roll gently up into a sitting position.
4. Lie on your stomach, a pillow under your abdomen, clasping hands behind your neck. Lift your trunk and hold for 10 seconds. It's easier if you have someone hold the lower half of your body steady by placing one hand in the small of your back and the other on your ankles.
5. Staying on your stomach, fold your arms under your head, keeping the pillow under your abdomen. Now lift your legs up, with your knees straight, and hold for 10 seconds. (Again, it is easier if someone holds your back steady with both hands.)

If you can do all these tests, you have good levels of muscular fitness and have sufficient strength and flexibility for your weight and height. However, if you failed even one of the tests, or had difficulty with them, you should consider yourself below par. You should work especially hard on the back exercise program described in Chapter 4 to get in better shape. Otherwise, the odds are high that you will suffer from back pain in the future.

Signs of a Disc Problem—Straight-Leg Tests
Lie on your back on a table or the floor, with your legs outstretched. Have someone place a hand under the heel of

your foot and gradually raise the leg, keeping it fully extended. If your knee automatically buckles and the leg bends when it is raised about halfway, or if pain is produced in either leg, there is a good chance that disc syndrome is present. If the ankle is bent by pushing the toes toward the head, thus stretching the nerve coming from the spine even further, and the pain becomes worse, it is even further confirmation of disc trouble, although there is still some chance the problem may be muscle spasm.

Sit on the edge of a table with both legs dangling, back as erect as possible and arms hanging at the sides. Have someone place a hand firmly on your thigh just above the knee. Have that person put his or her other hand under the heel of the same leg, and gradually straighten the leg by pushing the heel upward. Your partner should keep raising your leg upward slightly higher than the point of being level. If there is no problem, the leg should straighten out with no resistance or discomfort. If you tend to flip over backward or have to brace yourself with your hands to keep from falling back, you could have a disc problem. Test one leg, then the other.

Special Tests for Infants and Children

Gentle Tests for Infants

A thorough physical examination should be made by a doctor on every baby at birth, once every month for the first few months, and every three or six months after that. At each of these examinations, the doctor should check the child's muscles and bones to determine how they are developing. Meanwhile you can be alert at home for warning signs of trouble that should then be checked further with the doctor. You must do tests on infants *very* gently and carefully, never forcing motion.

19

- Compare the legs to make sure they are the same size and the same length.
- Check to see if there is any swelling, pain, redness, or heat at any place.
- Look for any tightness of the skin, especially around creases. All skin folds should move freely over the underlying bone or muscle.
- With the baby lying on his or her back, check the folds and creases of the thighs to see if they are equal and even. Turn the baby over on the stomach and check the creases in the back also.
- Place your hands around the baby's sides and hold the infant in the air. Check if the legs and feet hang normally and equally, or if one leg seems shorter or more bent than the other.
- If a child is old enough to stand or is walking, you can also check to see if the feet are turned outward or inward or if the feet and legs are spread wide apart as though needed for extra support. Also look carefully to see if the legs are extremely bowed, or if there is a sideways curve in the spine.

If you find any of these signs, call them to your doctor's attention. And if at any time your child complains of backache, especially at night, inform your doctor promptly. In children, this may sometimes be a symptom of a serious underlying disease.

Check a Child for Scoliosis
All children from age 8 on should be periodically screened for signs of spinal curvature, because if it is detected early, surgery can often be avoided.

Have the child strip to the waist. Carefully observe the

child's back while he or she stands erect, feet together, arms hanging relaxed. Check for the following:

- Shoulders at unequal levels
- Two sides of the hips uneven
- Waistline uneven
- Spine curved to one side
- One shoulder blade more prominent than the other

You can also check for curvature by putting ink marks on each of the vertebra and then see if the marks make a straight line or are crooked. Also have the child bend over, and see if there is a difference in level between the right and left side of the back or a hump on one side of the back.

If you find any of these signs, there is a possibility of scoliosis, and you should have your child examined as soon as possible by a doctor, and if necessary treatment can begin promptly.

Recent school screenings indicate that 10 to 12 percent of youngsters screened have this deformity to some extent. The curvature of the spine may appear gradually at first, and then may progress rapidly as the child grows older. If the curvature is not corrected before age 17 or 18, it may remain for the rest of a person's life. If it becomes severe, it can cause pain, lung damage, a hunched back, even death.

In adults, scoliosis can also be caused by degenerative arthritis of the spine. Mild curves in adults usually require no treatment but should be monitored to make sure they are not worsening.

For most child or teen-aged patients, some form of corrective brace, usually worn for about a year, sometimes only at night, is necessary to help the spine grow straight. A spinal pacemaker can also be used that gives electrical stimulation to the muscles on one side of the spine while the person sleeps.

There are a number of exercises that are helpful also (but all should be done under the guidance of a physician).

When to See Your Doctor

If any of these tests—whether in adults or children—indicates a possible abnormality, check with your physician so that he or she can investigate it further. In 90 percent of the cases, the weaknesses you found can be helped by the program we are going to outline for you, but in a few cases there could be some more serious underlying problem. You should have it checked out just to make sure that there is nothing to worry about. Read Chapter 10 to find out more about when and how to go to the doctor.

No matter what any of the at-home tests show, if you or any member of your family has frequent backaches, you should discuss the problem with your doctor and get his or her guidance.

CHAPTER THREE

When Your Back Hurts and You Need Help *Now*

What can you do right away when your back hurts—to ease your back when you have typed too long, overworked in the garden, or lifted too much furniture—and you need something you can do right away for first aid and fast relief?

Here are some instant helpers, easy techniques for quick relief as soon as your back starts hurting. Remember, however, that these techniques are only first aid measures for temporary relief. To keep painful attacks from happening again, to strengthen your back so that nagging aches now won't become excruciating pain later, you need to follow the entire Better Back Program outlined in the rest of the book.

The following are not back-*strengthening* exercises (we will give you these later). They are special techniques designed to relax your muscles and give relief when you are in the throes of an attack of back pain.

See which ones give you the most relief; then do them as many times a day as necessary to gain relief. Meanwhile, start the exercise program (Chapter 4), work on your body mechanics (Chapter 5), and if you are a smoker, stop smoking immediately. There are many theories as to why smoking makes a

difference in back pain, but we have definitely seen more back
pain in those who smoke.

Back Pain Relief Techniques You Can Do Yourself

Back Arching

If you have been working in a stooped position and find you
have difficulty straightening up or your back is starting to hurt,
then stand up, place your hands in the small of your back, and
bend backward five or six times, accentuating the curve in your
back to compensate the stooped-over curve it has been in.

Alternate Arch

Sitting or standing, put your arms behind your back at hip
level, clasping your hands together. Keep your arms straight,
squeeze your shoulder blades together as hard as you can, and
try to make your elbows touch. Hold to the count of 5. Relax
and wiggle your shoulders. This stretches muscles of the spine,
takes pressure off nerves, and relieves tension.

Back Flattening

Lie flat on your back with knees bent and feet flat on the
floor a foot or so from your buttocks. Pull in your abdominal
muscles; then tighten your buttock muscles so your back flattens
against the floor. Hold. Relax. Repeat 10 times. Relax again,
letting your back flatten against the floor. (Put a pillow under
your knees if you wish.)

Knee-Chest Pulls

In the same position, gently pull one knee up to your chest
with both hands. Do 10 times in little gentle pulls. Repeat with
the other leg 10 times. Try both knees together to see which
works better.

Lying Face Down

Although lying flat on your back is the traditional emergency way to ease an aching back, many people find that lying face down with arms at the side works better, putting an exaggerated curve into the back rather than flattening it. Do whichever makes you feel best. Either way, take deep breaths and let your back muscles relax.

If this worked well to relieve pain, then you may also try the same position, but propping yourself up on your forearms, which will arch your back further. If lying face down made your back hurt worse, discontinue that exercise and do not do the propping up on your forearms.

Yoga Stretch

Sit with your legs spread out in a V. Place the sole of one foot against the inner thigh of the other leg, and gently reach over the stretched-out leg as far as you can, stretching toward your toes. Hold for 30 to 60 seconds. This position stretches your hamstrings and muscles of the lower back, often relieving muscle spasms.

Leg Up

Lie on your back on the floor with your buttocks about 4 inches from a chair and your lower legs and feet resting on top of the chairseat. Use pillows, if you wish, under your head, or under your buttocks, and keep your buttocks close to the chair so that your knees are bent. Rest in this position and let your back flatten.

Help From a Slant Board

Lying feet up and head down on a slant board can help to straighten out the spine and flatten the back. This actually acts as a form of traction. In addition, muscles relax, sagging abdominal muscles get a lift, and any congestion or swelling are relieved in the legs.

You can buy a slant board or make one yourself by using any suitable large board (such as a door or a piece of plywood). Prop it up firmly on something so that your feet are a foot or so higher than your head.

Some people have good results producing this same traction effect hanging by their arms from a trapeze bar.

Lumbar Roll

Roll a towel into a long cylinder shape, lie on your back, and put the towel in the small of your back for support. Lie relaxed for 5 minutes or more.

The Tennis Ball Solution

After stretching and relaxing for a few minutes, put two tennis balls on the floor, and lie down on them so that they are under the small of your back, one on each side of your spine. Breathe deeply and slowly, relax all over, then slowly shift your body weight back and forth and work the balls around. You can use the tennis balls for a massage all over your back or just in the problem area that is bothering you.

Many people find that the tennis ball massage works for a painful hip also.

Try Heat

Heat can be very useful in easing discomfort and promoting relaxation. Almost any form of heat can be used—hot water bottle, heating pad, heat lamp, hot wet towel (wrapped in a dry towel to prevent scalding). If you use a heating pad, have it on for 20 to 30 minutes and turn it off for 20 to 30 minutes. Don't sleep with it on; it can heat up enough to burn your skin. Some people like to use a hydrocollator pack that you heat in water and then wrap in a towel. You can also have wet heat by soaking in a hot bath tub, or even better, a whirlpool. A shower works best if you wrap a towel around your back to hold the heat on your back while you shower.

Some doctors do not agree with applying heat to a sore back, but believe that if the muscles are inflamed, they are already congested, and heat might increase the blood and congestion in the area even more, which the muscle doesn't need.

Different people react in different ways, and there is only one way to find out how your body will react—test for yourself whether heat makes you feel better or worse.

Try Cold Applications

Cold in some people works better than heat, especially if there is muscle spasm. An ice rubdown often can help by returning the muscle to its relaxed state, eliminating the spasm. Sometimes it works best to use ice in the beginning, when there is inflammation or spasm, and then to apply heat later.

An at-home ice massage. Fill a paper cup with water and put it in the freezer until frozen. When ready to use, tear off the rim of the cup so some of the ice is exposed, leaving the bottom of the cup for holding. Massage the entire painful muscle area with the ice, using circular or up-and-down strokes. Do not hold the ice in one spot. There will be a cold sensation when the ice is first applied, then an aching, then after about 5 minutes, a burning sensation. At this point, stop for a minute or so; then massage with the ice again until the burning disappears and there is numbness. This is the crucial phase. Do not massage beyond the numbness stage or for more than 7 minutes in one area.

An alternative method is to fill a plastic bag, shower cap,

hot water bottle, or ice bag with ice cubes; wrap the ice-filled bag in a wet towel; and place it over the area, keeping it in place until numbness occurs (usually 20 to 30 minutes). Or use a bag of frozen vegetables that are handy in your freezer.

Repeat either procedure two to three times a day, or even every 2 hours. When pain is gone, you can gently exercise the area.

Have a Massage

An all-body massage plus a gentle massage of the local painful area can be helpful in reducing muscle spasm and promoting relaxation. The person giving the massage should use warm oil or warm rubbing alcohol or witch hazel and rub toward the heart. If pain eases enough, the person can rub more forcefully and knead gently to help loosen stiff muscles.

Try a Corset

A well-fitted corset 12 to 15 inches wide can sometimes give support and temporarily relieve discomfort. However, corsets should be worn only as a temporary measure and be discontinued as soon as acute pain is gone; then back-strengthening exercises should begin.

You May Have to Go to Bed and Stay There

If you have tried all the relaxing quick-fix techniques and your back still hurts a great deal, you may have strained a ligament and may have to stay in bed for the day, or even two, to take the strain off your back. (The old way of treating a bad back was with weeks or even months in bed. The most recent medical experience indicates that spending a long time in bed does far more harm than good, allowing muscles needed for recovery to atrophy.)

The best position in bed is lying flat on your back with a pillow under the knees. Another good position is to lie curled up on your side with a pillow between your knees to keep your spine from twisting.

Don't lie on a soft bed or lumpy sofa; choose the firmest mattress in your house, or have someone put the mattress on the floor.

The Most Important Thing to Remember

Whether your pain comes on gradually from being bent over at some job like painting or pulling weeds or instantly with a sudden stab from some usually innocent motion, the important thing is that you stay relaxed and calm.

Becoming tense or angry or starting to panic can cause your body to tighten up and aggravate the situation. Typically an attack of pain is followed by a muscle spasm, which in itself then causes pain. By staying relaxed and using the instant relief techniques described, it will help give you protection against the circle of pain and muscle spasm and more pain. If you ease the initial pain quickly enough, the spasm never occurs.

When to Call the Doctor

You should contact your doctor under the following circumstances:

- If the backache persists and gets no better.
- If backaches start occurring more frequently or severely.
- If you have other symptoms with the backache, such as fever, urinary problems, or genital symptoms.
- If pain radiates down an arm or leg.
- If pain wakes you up in the middle of the night.
- If you also have numbness or tingling in your arm or leg or a feeling of weakness.
- If the backache does not improve a little with a day of rest.
- If you are injured at work (a doctor's statement is required for Worker's Compensation).

Prevent More Back Pain Attacks

Again, these are only temporary measures for quick, instant relief. The best way to deal with back pain is to avoid it altogether by strengthening your back and learning how to take care of it, as we'll show you step by step in the following chapters.

CHAPTER FOUR

The Better Back Six-Week Exercise Program

Exercises are one of the most important phases of your program toward being free from any more back pain.

However, many exercise programs offer exactly the opposite of what the back needs; they often don't help the back at all, and, even more important, they may cause harm to the back. In fact, many patients have back problems caused by the very exercise programs they began supposedly to improve their fitness. Children can end up with back problems from improper calisthenics, and even old exercise standbys are surprisingly ineffective or even potentially dangerous if you have a weak back. Therefore, if you have problems with your back, be sure to follow only this program or one specifically recommended by your physician.

Exercises People with Back Problems Should Never Do

- Do not do traditional sit-ups.
- Do not do pull-ups or push-ups.
- Do not do back-bends to the floor, hip twists, backward trunk circling, or backward neck rolls.

- Do not touch your toes standing with your legs straight.
- Do not do donkey kicks (kicking up your legs while on hands and knees).
- Do not work out on parallel bars.
- Do not do long periods of jumping jacks or other jumping exercises that pound the joints.

All these exercises can do harm to your spine.

The Better Back Exercise Program

Our program has been designed to avoid these problems. We will be recommending only those exercises that have been found in clinical practice to work and not to do harm.

This is a graduated program, designed to be suitable for everyone, from small children to grandparents, whether in shape or not, because it begins at an easy level and can be adjusted so that you can always be at a level that is safe and comfortable for you, while you gain strength and improved function each day. (But even though the exercises are gentle, if you have any current or past back problems, you should check with your doctor before beginning the program to make absolutely sure that you do not have a special condition that should be treated in a different manner, or your doctor may want to modify the program to suit your particular needs.)

What makes our exercises different is that we want you to do them in slow motion. The newest research studies have shown some unexpected results: muscles that move slowly during exercise become stronger and in less time than do the same muscles moving quickly in the same exercise.

A common problem with back pain is that it can make you want to hold very still, since moving can be painful. However, not using muscles will, over time, cause them to lose range of motion and weaken, or they may shorten, tightening up and causing you to feel even more pain and stiffness. With the slow-motion exercises, you can break out of this pain barrier.

Another reason that the exercises work so well is that our program is planned around what has now become the exercise concept of the 1990s: cross-training. It incorporates exercises to increase flexibility, *plus* strength-training exercises, *plus* aerobic exercises. It strengthens your back muscles, and your abdominal and buttocks muscles, which results in increased support of your back and increased flexibility to the back and hips. It increases the flow of blood to your back. And, through the walking part of the program, it provides aerobic conditioning for your entire body.

The exercises that are part of the program have been so beneficial to the back that we have been using them in patients before back surgery to build up back strength and flexibility to make for a speedier recovery. Many times these exercises do so much good that patients with even the most severe pain and weakness *do not have to have the surgery that was scheduled!*

One woman, an aeronautical engineer from California who had had back pain that got worse and worse over several years after an accident, came to the Institute after three doctors had told her she would have to have surgery. After a diagnostic workup to determine the location and severity of the cause of her pain, she was entered into the physical therapy, diet, and exercise program. She turned out to be one of the lucky ones—after five weeks on the program, she had strengthened her muscles, which resulted in better support for her spine, increased her flexibility, and lost 12 pounds, thus taking a great deal of strain off the back. She was told to keep up the program and check in with us again in a month, or sooner if her pain started again. She continued the exercises, lost another 10 pounds, and was still pain-free at the end of the month. She never needed the surgery.

Many people, of course, still need surgery. This group gets the most benefit from exercise plus surgery. One woman was a dramatic example that we all like to remember. She had had seven operations—laminectomies (surgical removal of the posterior arch of a vertebra)—and could walk only with crutches. Now in addition to her back pain, her shoulders were becoming damaged and painful from the constant wear and tear of using the crutches. She gradually worked on our exercise and physical therapy program until she was doing quite well in both; then after this strengthening of her muscles we did surgery. After surgery she did more exercising and more therapy. For the first time in 10 years she was able to walk without crutches. She asked permission to sing at our Christmas party in appreciation for the results. It was the kind of success story that makes you want to stay in the field of medicine!

Of every 100 back patients who come into the Institute, about 40 are there because of an automobile or work accident or other acute injury, and about 60 are there with back pain that has been with them for years. All of them—after a careful diagnostic evaluation and medication when needed—go on the exercise and physical therapy program (unless their condition indicates bedrest or some other reason not to have exercise).

Of the patients with the acute problem, 40 percent report that their pain is gone in six weeks; in some of these there are recurrences, but in most the pain stays away. With three months of exercise and therapy, unless they had pain also going down their arms and legs, 90 percent of them report that their pain has gone away. In those who do have arm or leg pain with their back pain, 70 percent got better without surgery. In those whose pain does not go away or whose pain becomes worse or keeps recurring, we do surgery. After three months there is very little additional benefit from exercise in these acute cases.

Of the patients who come in with a chronic problem in which they have had their pain for years a much lower percentage have relief with just exercise and physical therapy. Their chances of not needing surgery is increased however if they also lose weight.

Even though you consider yourself to be physically fit, the exercises in our program should still be able to help you. You may be strong in general, but your back muscles may be weak. One famous tennis pro had severe back pain despite the fact that he played tennis seven days a week. Many times it is a matter of muscle *tightness* rather than muscle weakness that is the cause, which the exercises will also help.

Or it may be a protruding belly that is putting strain on your back. Weak abdominal muscles can mean added stress on the back muscles, so that strengthening abdominal muscles is very important in conquering back pain. Regular exercise also helps trim off any back-breaking extra pounds that you may be carrying around your middle.

(However, be on your guard. It is often recommended that abdominal muscles be strengthened by doing sit-ups with the legs stretched out straight. This is wrong. Traditional sit-ups mostly strengthen the hip flexors, which most people don't need, and they often cause overstress on the back and intense pressure on the lumbar discs.)

General exercise, especially walking, is also an important part of the program because of all the benefits from aerobic exercise. In addition, the kind of weight-bearing exercises that we recommend have been shown to increase density of bone, thus strengthening your back from within.

As part of the program at the GCOC Institute, we schedule walks for fitness every morning at a local shopping mall. We call it the Stride Inside Club. Walkers get their exercise by striding the corridors of the mall between 9 and 10 A.M. before the stores open for business. A physician and physical therapist supervise the walkers, assist them with warm-up exercises, answer questions, and do blood pressure tests before and after the walks. It provides a lot of fun and competition—walkers record the number of miles they have walked and their blood pressure readings and compare the results—and hundreds of people have signed up.

Exercise Timetable

The Better Back Exercise Program starts at a very easy level, slowly and gently easing your back muscles into good condition without danger. At first, the exercises may seem so easy that you may think they are not doing any good, but do not be tempted to skip the preliminary easy exercises. Your back will appreciate it.

When each new exercise is introduced, do it only a few times; then build up each day, doing the exercise more times and holding the various positions for longer periods. If an exercise is difficult for you, work at it for another week if necessary. If the exercise is easy for you, you can speed up your progress. In other words, move along at your own pace.

To get the maximum benefit, you should do the exercises every day for the six weeks. Later, you can reduce the frequency to every other day. Remember, anybody can do these exercises, no matter how old or how weak. One person may not be able to advance as far as another, but every single person will benefit to some extent. In a few weeks you will be amazed that anything so simple could have accomplished so much.

If You Think You Are Too Tired to Exercise

Contrary to what most people think, moderate exercising when you are tired at the end of the day can actually perk you up and make you feel better, and in fact it usually works well to counteract chronic fatigue, the kind of fatigue that drags you down day after day for long periods. If, however, you are unusually exhausted or are coming down with an illness, you should put off exercising for the next day or so.

If for some reason you stop exercising for several weeks, you should start at the beginning again so that your body will build back up gradually without strain. If you miss the exercises for only a few days, then you can back up just a little in the program.

The Results Will Come Fast

Within two or three weeks you should begin to see some results in the way you feel; you should have more energy, less pain, and more flexibility. By six weeks, you should see increased function and dramatic reduction in pain. Don't be impatient. Think in terms of the total six weeks. The way you feel then will have made it worthwhile. Remember, it took years to get your back the way it is; you can't change it in just a few days. You want an improvement that is safe and will last for the rest of your life.

Keep the program up for the full six weeks and you may never want to quit. You'll feel so good you will wonder how you were able to drag around as you were before.

Many patients like to use a chart like the one on the following page to keep track of their progress.

Important Do's and Don'ts

Do the exercises every day for maximum benefit and quickest results.

Set aside a specific time in your day for the exercises so that you do them regularly. Some people prefer to do them first thing in the morning; others prefer to relax with them after

Progress Chart

DATE						
Wall Stand						
Sponge						
Pelvic Tilt						
Pelvic Raise						
Single-Knee Raise						
Knee-Nose Touch						
Double-Knee Raise						
Single-Leg Raise						
Head-and-Shoulder Lift						
Little Leg Raise						
SPECIAL EXERCISES						
Lying Face Down						
Half Lift						
Whole Lift						
Easy Backbend						
Mad Cat/Old Horse						

Record your progress weekly

0 = Unable to do
1 = Able to do only a few times
2 = Able to do but with slight difficulty
3 = Able to do with ease

work before fixing dinner. You can do the exercises at any time of day (but not until an hour after eating).

Exercise on a firm (but not cold) surface. Most people like to use an exercise mat or a comforter on the floor for a little extra padding.

Exercise with bare feet in loose comfortable clothes. Put on some nice soft music to go with your slow-motion relaxed movements or, if you prefer, enjoy relaxing silence.

Do the warm-up exercises before you begin the more vigorous exercises. This gives your muscles time to adjust and loosen up.

Do each exercise slowly and smoothly. Remember: slow motion. Be relaxed. Don't use jerky movements. Do not hold your breath. Breathe easily and naturally.

When doing your exercises, hold the position for the prescribed time, slowly release each movement, and repeat each maneuver the prescribed number of times.

Don't skip any of the exercises unless they cause pain. If at any time you don't feel you are ready to advance to the next level, simply repeat that week's exercises for another week until you feel ready to progress. Doing a few exercises well will produce more results than will doing a large number poorly. Every day your muscles will be getting stronger, and more flexible, and the exercises will become easier and easier. When the more difficult exercises are introduced, your muscles will have been prepared by the exercising you did previously.

If at any time you have pain or significant discomfort or a peculiar sensation of any kind while doing any of the exercises, stop that exercise for several days. Try it again a few days later carefully and with fewer repetitions. If you still have discomfort, check with your doctor and get his or her approval before continuing. Demonstrate how the pain arises. Your doctor or physical therapist may be able to redesign the exercise for you.

Think about your muscles as you exercise. Feel them

becoming more relaxed, looser, more flexible. Feel how your back and entire body are beginning to work for you and how you are developing more natural movements and grace.

When you start your walking program, keep checking yourself to make sure your body is not pitched forward, which can strain you back. Do not slump; stand tall, and let your hips swing freely.

WARNING:

If you have back problems, don't do *any* exercises that are not part of this program without checking with your doctor first.

And most important, do not force your body into painful positions, *ever*. Any uncomfortable position should be worked on gradually without force and only with the approval of your doctor.

Six Weeks to a Better Back

Week One

Exercise 1. The Wall Stand Stand with your back to a wall or door, with your feet a few inches from the wall. Bend your knees, flatten your spine against the wall as much as you can, stretch your head up and your shoulders back and down. There will be some natural curve, but you shouldn't feel swaybacked. Keep trying to flatten your spine against the wall, and slide yourself back up. Hold flat against the wall in a standing position to a count of 5. (By the end of the week hold to 20.) Do 5 times.

Exercise 2. The Sponge Lie on your back on the floor. Take a slow deep breath, hold it. Feel any tension in your muscles. Let your breath go and the tension go. Let your entire body relax; let your arms and legs and jaw sag, limp and relaxed. Wobble your neck, shoulders, arms, legs, and feet to loosen them up. Raise both arms slowly and let them drop. Take a deep breath and exhale slowly. Let your body feel heavy; let your arms and legs go limp against the floor. Breathe slowly again. Slowly lift your shoulders toward your ears, then let them go. Lie quietly for several moments, relaxed and breathing slowly.

Exercise 3. The Pelvic Tilt   Still lying on your back, bend your knees and slide your feet about 12 inches toward you. Keep them flat on the floor and your arms loose at your sides or resting on your chest or abdomen. This is a basic position you will use for many of your back exercises. Contract your muscles to pinch your buttocks together, hold to the count of 5. Relax. Now contract your abdominal muscles and hold to the count of 5. Relax. (Do 5 times the first day, building up to 20 times each by the end of the week.)

In the same position, tighten your buttocks muscles and abdominal muscles at the same time (if you have difficulty tightening the buttocks and abdominal muscles at the same time, tighten your buttocks muscles first, then your abdominal muscles). You will feel the small of your back press against the floor. If you don't, try to push the small of your back down so it does go flat against the floor. Hold for a count of 5 the first day; build to a count of 20 by the end of the week. Repeat 5 times.

Whenever You Think About It...   Whenever you are sitting at your desk, watching television, waiting for a bus— whatever—tense your buttocks muscles and your abdomen and hold for a few seconds. Work at keeping your posture erect by thinking of your wall-stand exercise.

General Exercise   To increase your general fitness, take a walk for about 15 minutes every day this week.

Week Two

Do the Wall Stand for a count of 20.

Do the Sponge.

Do the Pelvic Tilt for a count of 20.

Add Exercise 4. The Pelvic Raise This is sometimes called the *Bridging Exercise*. Lie on your back on the floor with knees bent and feet flat. Contract your buttocks muscles and abdominal muscles to flatten your back to the floor. While the buttocks are squeezed and the abdomen held in, raise the buttocks slightly from the floor. Hold to a slow count of 5. Relax. By the end of the week, try to be able to hold the position to the count of 20.

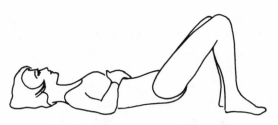

THE PELVIC TILT AND THE PELVIC RAISE

Add Exercise 5. The Single-Knee Raise Lie flat on your back on the floor in a pelvic tilt position with both knees bent. Grasp under your right knee with both hands and slowly bring it up as near to your chest as it will go without causing pain or discomfort. Hold to the count of 5. Slowly return leg to starting position. Repeat with left leg. Relax. Repeat 5 times for each leg.

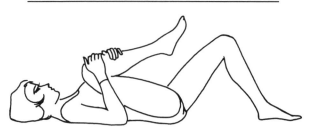

THE SINGLE KNEE RAISE

Whenever You Think About It... Keep doing the butt-belly contractions. Whether sitting, standing, or lying down, keep reminding yourself during the day to sit and stand up straight without letting yourself slouch. Practice standing tall with your head balanced and your abdomen sucked in.

General Exercise Continue walking every day, increasing your time to 20 to 30 minutes each day.

Week Three

Do the Wall Stand, the Sponge, and the Pelvic Tilt from Week One, for a count of 20. Do the Pelvic Raise and the Single-Knee Raise from Week Two, holding for a count of 20.

Add Exercise 6. The Knee-Nose Touch Lie on your back in the pelvic tilt position with both knees bent. With both hands under your right knee, bring your knee up as close to your head as is comfortable and bring your head forward until you can touch your nose or chin to your knee. Hold for as long as comfortable. Slowly drop your head back to the floor. Relax. Repeat with the right leg. Relax. Do each leg 5 times.

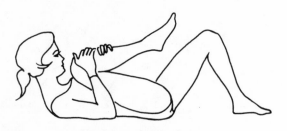

THE KNEE-NOSE TOUCH

Whenever You Think About It... Go barefoot whenever you are on soft surfaces like grass, carpeting, or at the beach. It strengthens muscles of your legs and feet. When you watch television sit cross-legged on the floor for a while. It increases flexibility of the hip.

General Exercise Continue your walking program. Increase your pace from a leisurely one to a brisk one. You want to get your walking up to an aerobic level so that it elevates the heart rate. Use the "talk" test: you should walk fast enough to make you breathe hard, but you should still be able to talk without gasping. If you can't talk easily, slow down a little.

Week Four

Do the Wall Stand, the Sponge, and the Pelvic Tilt. Do the Pelvic Raise and Single-Knee Raise for a count of 20. Do the Knee-Nose Touch.

Add Exercise 7. The Double-Knee Raise Lie on the floor on your back with knees bent and feet flat. Grasp under both knees with your hands and slowly pull them toward your chest. Let your pelvis lift; feel your spine touch the floor. Hold for 5 seconds (20 by the end of the week). Return to starting position. Relax. Do 5 times.

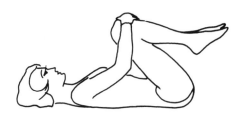

THE DOUBLE KNEE RAISE

Whenever You Think About It... When you wake up or when you are stretched out on a couch watching television, raise one leg a few inches, keeping the leg straight and the toes pointed toward your head. Alternate raising each leg as high as you want as many times as you want.

General Exercise You may continue your brisk walking for 30 minutes or more everyday, or you may begin a more vigorous sport such as swimming, cross-country skiing, or dancing. Whatever you choose, begin gradually. At first only swim for a few laps or dance half an hour. If you are a beginner at a sport, take lessons from a professional instructor to develop proper skills.

Week Five
Do the Wall Stand, the Sponge, the Pelvic Tilt, the Pelvic Raise, the Single-Knee Raise, the Knee-Nose Touch, and the Double-Knee Raise.

Add Exercise 8. The Single-Leg Raise Lie on your back with your arms in a comfortable position. Bend your left leg with your foot flat on the floor, and have your right leg extended straight. Keeping your right leg straight, raise it as high as you comfortably can. (Remember that you should be doing exercises in slow motion.) Hold the leg up for a count of 5. Slowly lower it to the floor. Relax. Repeat with the left leg. You will probably feel a pull in your hamstring muscles. In fact, many people have such tight, short hamstrings that they can only raise their legs halfway. Only raise your leg as far as is comfortable. Repeat 5 times. If you have any down-the-leg pain of sciatica, do not do this exercise.

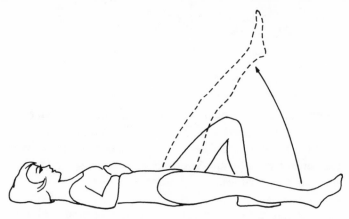

THE SINGLE LEG RAISE

Add Exercise 9. The Head-And-Shoulder Lift   Also called the Partial Sit-up. Lie on the floor on your back in the Pelvic Tilt position with your knees bent and your feet flat. You can either let your arms lie relaxed along your sides, or you can grasp your shoulders with your hands, whichever is more comfortable. Slowly raise your head and shoulders off the floor, flexing as far as you comfortably can. (It's like the knee-nose touch, but you are lifting your shoulders also.) Do not jerk, but raise yourself slowly. Try to hold for a count of 5. Slowly lower your head and shoulders and relax. Do 5 times. If you have weak abdominal muscles, this may be a difficult exercise for you, but continue and strengthen these muscles until you can do this exercise. You can vary this exercise by curling your right shoulder toward your left knee 5 times, and then curling your left shoulder toward your right knee 5 times.

Whenever You Think About It . . .   Put your arms behind your back, clasping your hands together. Keep your arms straight,

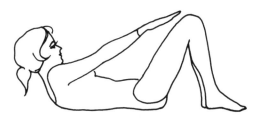

THE HEAD AND SHOULDER LIFT

and squeeze your shoulder blades together as hard as you can. Hold for a few seconds. Relax and wiggle your shoulders. When you are talking on the telephone or waiting for the water to boil or whatever, put your right foot up on a table or desk, keeping your leg straight. Gently lower your body toward your foot, reaching several times for the foot with your right hand. Repeat with left leg. Keep back straight, not swayback.

General Exercise Whether you are just walking or have taken up a sport, by now you should be feeling so much better that you will automatically be increasing your pace and time just because it feels so good and is enjoyable. Invite some other people to join you in your sport or your walking to make it even more fun and to help keep you on track. Make arrangements for all of you to meet on a regular schedule.

Week Six
Do the Wall Stand, the Sponge, the Pelvic Tilt, the Pelvic Raise, the Single-Knee Raise, the Knee-Nose Touch, the Double-Knee Raise, the Single-Leg Raise, and the Head-and-Shoulder Lift.

Add Exercise 10. On-Your-Back Little Leg Raise Lie on your back with your legs extended straight out, your arms along your sides or under your head, whichever is more comfortable for you. With your legs together, raise them very slowly 2 to 4 inches, no more. Do not arch your back. Hold for a count of 2 (later 5). Lower your legs slowly to the floor. Relax. Repeat 5 times. If you have difficulty, begin by doing one leg at a time for a few days and then doing both legs together.

Whenever You Think About It ... When you get out of the shower or bath, stand straight, grab a bath towel at each end, and hold it in front of you at arm's length. Keeping arms straight, raise towel overhead, then bring it down behind your back as far as you can, keeping elbows straight and towel stretched. Do as many times as you feel like it.

General Exercise Reward yourself. You have completed six weeks of great exercise and should be feeling more fit than you have in years. Buy yourself a present as lavish as you feel you can afford, a new tennis racket, a new swimming suit, even a week's vacation to enjoy your new body and show it off.

Special Exercises for the Person with a Disc Problem

For most people the exercises we have described are the most effective in strengthening the back and achieving a normal spinal curve, a "neutral" spine as orthopedic doctors call it. However, the person who has pain caused by disc problems or the person with osteoporosis often does well with what are called "extension" exercises. These exercises are designed for people whose backs feel better when they are lying on their stomachs with their backs arched rather than on their backs with their backs flat.

You may want to try these exercises to see how they work for you. If they cause pain, discontinue them, since certain medical conditions can be aggravated by extension. At GCOC we have found them very beneficial for patients with disc problems. Researchers at the Mayo Clinic also found some of them very helpful to a group of women with osteoporosis. Do Exercises 1 and 2 to start, then add the other three. Begin gradually and work up in number and intensity just as in the other exercises in this chapter. Usually back-*flattening* exercises which are the ten we previously described, are helpful for muscle strain or overuse, while the *extensor* exercises that follow are helpful for disc problems. If you are not sure which exercises are best for you, consult your doctor.

Extensor Exercise 1. Lying Face Down Lie face down with your arms beside your body and your head turned to one side. Breathe deeply and slowly. Relax for several minutes. Do this relaxing exercise each time before you do the other extension exercises.

Extensor Exercise 2. The Half Lift Start in a face-down position, then raise up and lean on your forearms. Stay in this position for a count of at least 20 as long as there is no pain.

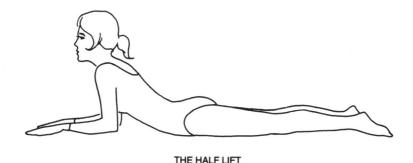

THE HALF LIFT

Extensor Exercise 3. The Whole Lift From the same face-down position, place your hands palms down on the floor under your shoulders. Straighten your arms and push the top half of your body up as far as it is comfortable. Let your hips and legs hang relaxed and let your lower back sag. Hold for a second or two, and then return to the starting position. Do 5 times. Each time you do this exercise, try to raise yourself a little higher, but always letting your legs and hips stay on the floor.

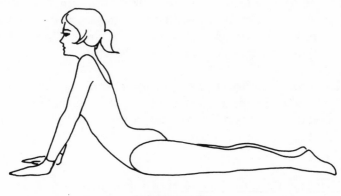

THE WHOLE LIFT

Extensor Exercise 4. The Easy Backbend Stand upright with your feet slightly apart, place your hands in the small of your back. Bend backward at the waist as far as you comfortably can. (But don't arch your neck.) Hold for a second or two and return to the starting position. Do 5 times. This is a good exercise to do to get a "neutral" spine again when you are doing stooping work such as gardening. Try to do it frequently as you work, before pain starts.

Extensor Exercise 5. Mad Cat, Old Horse This exercise comes from Sweden. Start on the floor on your hands and knees, with the knees comfortably spread, the hands palms down on the floor directly under the shoulders, and the eyes looking ahead. Slowly arch up your back like a cat that has just seen an enemy. Hold for a few seconds, then slowly let your back down until it's sagging like that of an old horse. Keep your

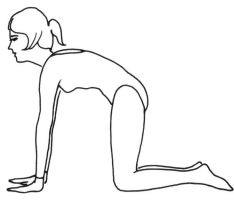

THE MAD CAT

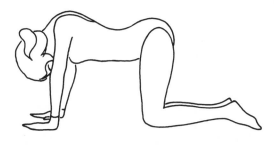

THE OLD HORSE

head down or straight ahead, but do not arch your neck. Repeat 5 times. Now bring your hands closer to your knees and repeat the same movements to exercise a different part of the spine.

Special Pool Exercises

If you have access to a swimming pool, exercising in water is a gentle low-impact way to exercise the joints and muscles. The buoyancy of the water supports your body and lessens stress on the joints. (In chest-deep water you weigh only about 10 percent of your on-land weight, so if you weigh 150 pounds, you have only about 15 pounds to carry around in the water.) You can do things in the water that you couldn't do on solid ground.

Swimming exercises are an important part of the program at GCOC. Almost all of the patients come to the pool for exercises whether or not they have surgery, and if they have surgery, they begin the pool exercises the third week after surgery as part of their back-strengthening program.

Water provides resistance as you move your body and limbs, helping you build muscle strength. It has the effect of using ankle and wrist weights when you push against the water.

Exercising in a warm pool is especially beneficial because there is an increase in blood supply to the muscles, in metabolism, and in respiratory rate, and a decrease in blood pressure. We keep the GCOC pool between 92 and 96 degrees Fahrenheit. (Note: During an attack of back pain you should avoid swimming in water below 70 degrees Fahrenheit and should take a hot shower after swimming to avoid getting chilled.)

When first entering a pool, relax and enjoy the soothing water. When your muscles and joints feel more comfortable and relaxed, slowly begin your exercise routine. Allow enough time after exercising to again relax muscles before getting out of the water.

When you do your water exercises, move slowly and gently. Follow through complete joint range of motion if possible, but do not force movement. Stop if you experience any sudden or increased pain.

Do 5 to 10 repetitions, as much as can be tolerated. Pain that lasts for more than 1 to 2 hours after exercise may indicate overexertion. Cut back next time.

Any individuals who have severe joint damage or joint replacement should check with their doctor or surgeon before doing any of these exercises.

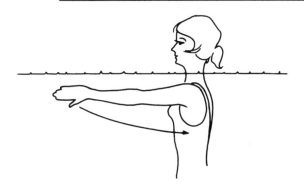

PUSH

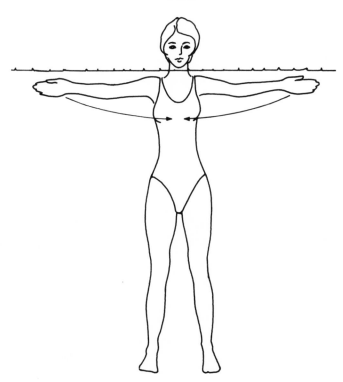

PULL

1. *Push and pull.* Stand with feet apart. Extend arms in front of you with the back of your hands touching, thumbs pointing down. Push against the water and move your arms behind your back as quickly as you can. Face palms forward, thumbs pointing up, and repeat back to in front of you with a pulling motion.
2. *Torso stretch.* Stand with your left side to the wall of the pool and hold onto the wall with your left hand. Stretch up

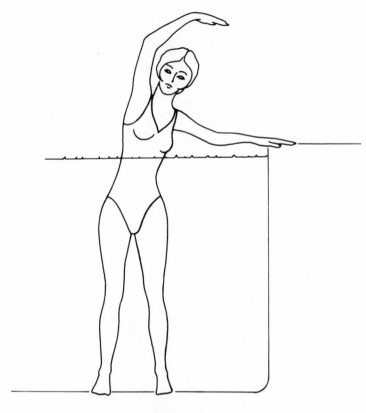

TORSO STRETCH

with your other arm and reach high overhead and toward the wall. Switch sides and repeat.

3. *Leg swing.* Again hold onto the wall of the pool with one hand. Keeping knees straight, lift right leg slowly forward to a comfortable height, hold for a count of 5, then slowly swing leg backward. Keep upper body straight. Keep motion in the hip, not the waist.

4. *Side-leg lift.* Stand with your left side to the pool wall, with left hand on the wall for balance. With knees relaxed, swing right leg out toward center of pool and back. Keep

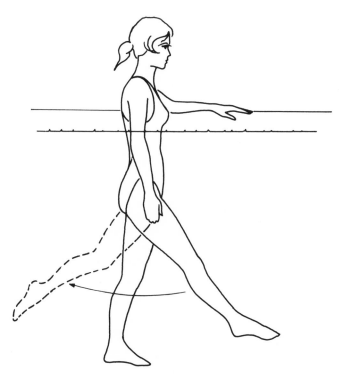

THE LEG SWING

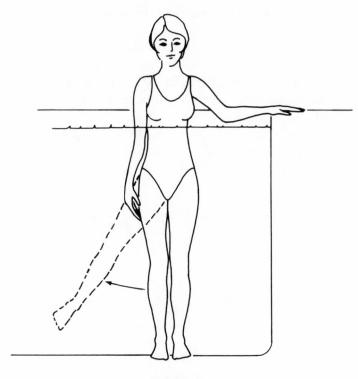

THE SIDE LEG LIFT

your toes and your kneecaps pointed straight ahead. Repeat with other leg.

5. *Straight-back kick.* Hold on to the side of the pool with both hands, body outstretched on water and kick, keeping the back straight. For variety, you can use a kickboard, putting it under your chest for support so your back is not overly arched.

6. *Pool walking.* Do walking in the pool as though you were on land. First, walk normally in shoulder-deep water, with long steps and swinging your arms. Then "march," leaning

slightly forward, pulling in your stomach muscles, lifting knees high and pumping your arms.

7. *Backstroke.* Do the backstroke each time you are in the pool, for whatever length of time you are comfortable with, gradually building up to longer distances.

Spa Exercises

If you are fortunate enough to have a home spa, it can provide the warmth, massage, and buoyancy needed for many water exercises. Soaking in the hot water allows muscles to become relaxed, which can then make it especially easy to perform exercises.

However, since there isn't enough room for most of the exercises, do only what you can. For example, you can do knee-to-chest raises while sitting in the spa or little leg raises. The size and shape of the spa will determine the types of exercises that you can do.

Consider that you may need help getting in and out of the spa. Someone should be nearby for help if necessary, especially the first few times.

Check the thermometer for appropriate temperature before entering the spa. Different people react differently to heat; therefore, anyone who feels lightheaded or nauseated should get out of the water immediately. If you are exercising, keep the heat around 96 or 97 degrees Fahrenheit; if you are not exercising, it is okay to go higher.

Latest reports indicate that if you are pregnant you should not use a spa. Also consult with your doctor before using a spa or pool if you have any special medical conditions, especially lung or heart disease, circulatory problems, high or low blood pressure, diabetes, multiple sclerosis, thyroid disease, or skin irritations.

Never use a spa or pool while or after using alcohol or

drugs. These may cause sleepiness or drowsiness or may raise or lower blood pressure.

If you are overweight, have severe arthritis, or for other reasons are unsure on your feet, you may find it a good idea to install grab rails or steps for getting in and out of the spa or pool.

Maintenance for the Future

Your back should now be stronger and feel better than it ever has before, and it is important that you don't let it return to a poor condition. This maintenance program is designed to keep your good condition and to prevent future problems.

You now need to do only a few exercises to keep up the strengthening you have done over the six weeks, and so the maintenance program takes only a few minutes each day. Most people like to do their exercises in the morning before they have started the day, sometimes while still in bed.

Do the exercises in the program that made you feel especially good or that especially helped your back. The ones that are most effective for most people are the Pelvic Tilt (Exercise 3), the Pelvic Raise (Exercise 4), the Double-Knee Raise (Exercise 7), the Head-and-Shoulder Lift (Exercise 9), and the On-Your-Back Little Leg Raise (Exercise 10).

After the exercises, rest for a few moments in the basic pelvic tilt position, and you should be ready for a great day.

For your maintenance and prevention program, you may if you wish do the exercises every day, but you don't have to—three or four times a week is fine.

Keep these maintenance exercises going. If you have started this program because you had a back problem, don't think that once your pain and stiffness have disappeared you can do without the exercises. If you continue to do them and follow your doctor's other instructions, your back could possibly be strong and pain-free for life. But if you stop doing the exercises, your back pain may return.

Also as part of your maintenance program, and to protect against possible future trouble, you should continue to do the Pelvic Tilt and any of the whenever-you-think-about-it exercises from the program that you thought especially helpful.

If you would like to do your exercising with a video, we have found Dr. Art Ulene's *Back Pain Relief* video accurate and easy to follow, as well as Dr. David Lehrman's back exercise video.

CHAPTER FIVE

Redesigning Your Body Mechanics—
How to Sit, Stand, Walk, Drive, Lift,
Make Love, Carry, and Sleep for a
Better Back

When you walk into the lobby of the Gulf Coast Orthopedic Center you are surrounded by mirrors. In fact almost every hallway and public room is covered with mirrors—floor to ceiling and wall to wall. It gives you a strange feeling at first to see yourself everywhere, but it serves its purpose well—you see yourself at every turn, how you stand and how you walk. With every look, you are reminded to stand tall and sit erect. The downside is that patients aren't very pleased with what they see when they first come in. The upside is how happy they are at their posture and energetic bearing when they are free of pain and standing tall after having been through the program.

Faulty posture and improper body mechanics are two common underlying causes of back pain. They can alter the curve of the back and put severe stress on back muscles and ligaments. If you have rounded shoulders, a slumped back, or a protruding abdomen, if you walk incorrectly, sit slumped, and lift things improperly, you probably already have back pain, or you may have it in the future.

But you are also headed for trouble if you have an exaggerated, military stance with shoulders thrown too far back, chest and buttocks sticking out, and a huge swayed curve to the back. That, too, means backache.

The advice in this section will give you the proper techniques for good body mechanics—techniques to train your body back into proper balance, so that your head, rib cage, and pelvis are stacked up correctly, and you have a smooth bearing and efficient body motion, all of which reduce the risk of stress and injury to your back.

Redesigning Your Body Mechanics

Check Your Posture

1. Stand in front of a full-length mirror in your underwear. Check how you look when you stand in your usual posture. Are you saggy and slumped? Do you stand with a forced military position? Does your abdomen stick out? Are you swaybacked? See the figure on page 16.

2. Stand with your back against a wall with your head and shoulders touching the wall and your heels about 2 inches from the wall. Try to make your back as flat as possible. You should just barely be able to slide your hand between the wall and the small of your back, not your fist. If not, then your posture needs work.

3. Face the wall with toes touching the wall. Slowly lean in to the wall, keeping your normal posture. Notice which part of your body touches first. If your chest touches first, your posture is probably good. If your abdomen touches first, your posture is very poor and your back is under a great deal of strain.

Note when testing children. Young children often have a natural potbelly, and from age 6 to 12 they may have swayback,

61

slightly rounded shoulders, and a flat chest, so do not let these variations worry you. By the adolescent years, however, the abdomen should be flat, and the normal adult posture should have been attained.

How to Have Better Posture

There are five basic things that you need to remember about good posture and body mechanics. Remind yourself of them throughout the day until they are second nature.

1. All day, in everything you do, try to stand tall.
2. Keep your head straight, not thrust forward or looking down. You should feel that your head is just balancing on top of the spine.
3. Pull your stomach in. Starting at your pubic bone, imagine you are "zipping up" your abdominal muscles.
4. Pull your buttocks in and your pelvis up.
5. Avoid swayback.

After you have tried these tricks, go back and do the posture tests again and see how you look now in the mirror. Doesn't your good posture make you look much better than you did before?

Exercises to Improve Posture

Do these exercises when you get up from bed and whenever else you can during the day.

1. Stand with your heels and shoulders to the wall, as you did in the posture test, and rhythmically push the small of your back toward the wall to make less space between it and the wall. Squeeze your buttocks in and pull your abdomen in—feel your back flatten out, just as it does in the Pelvic

Tilt exercise you are doing in the exercise program. Relax the shoulders. Try walking around the room in this position. For correct standing and walking posture, you should maintain this pelvic tilt all the time. Return to the wall and flatten your back again. Do 5 times.

2. Stand with your feet slightly apart and touch the tips of your fingers together in front of your chest; your elbows should be at shoulder height. Keeping your elbows bent, thrust your upper arms back and tighten your shoulder blades (to the count "1–2"). Be sure your head is not thrust forward. Straighten your arms and swing them back at shoulder height, with your thumbs pointing toward the ceiling (to the count "3–4"). Do 5 times.

3. Make a windmill action with your arms. Stand straight (again, be sure your head is not thrust forward), bring one arm forward, then up, then back and down. Keep your shoulders back as much as you can and make large, free-swinging circles. Do 20 times with right arm, then 20 times with the left.

Posture Games

1. Imagine that your head is a balloon, trying to pull your body up, and that your spine is a string attached to it.
2. Imagine you are carrying water with a yoke over your shoulders and two buckets.
3. Pretend you are a puppet suspended from a string in the ceiling.

How to Sit Down and Get Up

To get into a chair, start with the backs of the legs touching the chair, and lower yourself to the edge of the chair. Slide back into the chair and let your back relax into the chair.

To get out of a chair, slide to the edge of the chair. With chin tucked under slightly, straighten your knees and lift yourself out of the chair with your legs. With an armchair, also use your arms to push yourself up.

How to Sit Without Tiring Your Back

The pressure per square inch on a spinal disc is about twice as great when sitting as when standing. People who sit all day usually have a very high incidence of back pain. But sitting properly, moving about between sitting periods, and exercising daily will help most of these people prevent the pain.

You can sit properly in two ways: one, sitting back in your chair with your lower back supported, or two, sitting straight, away from the back of the chair, with a slight curve in your back but not a swayback.

If a chair that you have does not provide proper support, you may want to purchase a back support, such as a lumbar roll, a cylinder-shaped foam cushion 4 to 5 inches in diameter that fits between the chair and the small of your back.

To put less strain on your back, especially if a chair is too high, put one or both feet up on a low stool, with your knees bent. (A good trick when sitting at a desk is to slide out the bottom drawer and rest one or two feet on it.)

Especially when reading or sewing, don't thrust your head forward or drop your head on your chest, which strains your neck. Don't slump or slouch. If you have your weight on your tailbone, it may get tender or painful.

When working at a desk, bend forward from the hips, not the waist. Have things close to you so you do not have to reach far forward on your desk to work.

In recliner chairs, if you sit upright instead of with the recliner pushed back, be careful that the thick padding under the head does not force your head and neck forward, causing strain.

Use a rocking chair occasionally. It helps relax back muscles and tends to counteract a slouch or swayback posture.

Sit on the floor sometimes in the "Indian position." It's an excellent way to watch television (better than in bed with your neck bent!). For centuries the Japanese, who sat on mats on the floor, almost never had back problems, but as they have adopted Western ways, including sitting on chairs, backaches are becoming more frequent.

If your back gives you trouble when sitting on bleacher seats or other backless benches, you might try a portable sling called a Nada Chair. It consists of a cushion that fits behind your back and two loops that fit around your knees, with the reverse pressure helping to hold your back erect.

Most important, move around occasionally as you work. Stand up and walk around every half hour or so.

Instant Relief when Your Back Is Tired from Sitting

1. Lean forward in your chair and lower your head to your knees for 2 to 3 minutes. This tends to counteract any arched curve in your back that you may have acquired. Or if your problem is that you are slouching, stand up and bend backward five or six times and walk around a few minutes. The important thing is to move around at regular intervals *before* any pain starts.

2. If you find your neck or shoulder muscles starting to tighten and bunch up from being in one position, lace your fingers behind your head, and gently push arms backward as far as you can. Hold as long as comfortable. This will help stretch and loosen tight shoulder muscles.

3. Stand in a doorway, placing your hands approximately shoulder high on both sides of the door jamb, your feet about 18 inches apart. Slowly more forward into the open doorway, without letting your back arch. Your chest will be

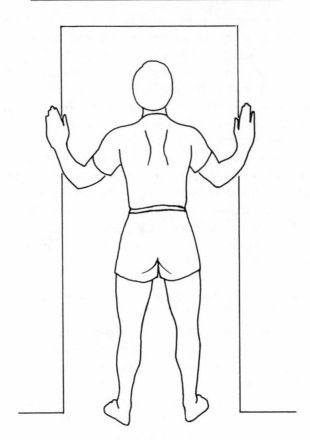

THE DOORWAY STRETCH

pushed forward and your shoulder blades will come togeth-er. It's a good muscle stretch.

Additional Ways of Ensuring Good Posture

Choosing a Chair to Help Your Back
The fanciest, most expensive chair isn't always the best for

your back. The important thing in choosing a chair is to find one that helps keep the back almost flat or just slightly rounded.

Chairs that usually support the back best are the classic rocker with a straight back, the Breuer-type tubular steel and cane chair, and a reclining chair (sitting back in a good recliner is like being on your back with your knees propped up).

The front-to-back depth of a chair seat should allow your knees to bend comfortably when you're sitting straight against the chair back. It should be low enough so that you can place both feet on the floor, but not so low that rising from it is difficult.

If you use the chair at a desk, you should be able to pull that chair close to the desk. Avoid chair arms that prevent your getting in close, making you hunch forward. (However, if you are not at a desk, a chair with arms makes it possible to rest your forearms on the chair and allow the muscles of the upper back to be relaxed.)

For typing or working at a computer, the chair should be adjustable so that you can move the padded back up or down to give firm support to the center of your back. You also should adjust the seat up or down so that you do not have to reach up to the keyboard, nor hunch over to peer down at it; keys should be about waist high. When you lean back in the chair, it should give a little, but not much.

When you buy a chair, try to find furniture scaled to your size. Ask to have a one-week trial to take the chair home and test it. If your back is uncomfortable in the chair, or numbness, stiffness, or pain appears in the feet, legs, shoulders, or neck, the chair is not right for you. Take it back.

How to Choose Shoes That Are Best for Your Back

Your feet can often be at the bottom of a back problem. When your feet are weak, or improperly balanced, or if they hurt, they can throw the legs, hips, and eventually the back out of balance.

When you buy shoes, make sure the sole is flexible (bend it to see); the shank or arch support should *not* bend. The leather should be soft with no ridges, wrinkles, or bumps inside to rub. Make sure shoes are wide enough (about ¼ inch bigger than your foot, loose enough so that a little bit of leather can be pinched.)

Avoid sling-backs that slip and very high heels that pitch the body forward. (As the height of women's shoes goes up, so does the incidence of foot and back problems.) Often a woman can get rid of back pain simply by switching to a more reasonable medium heel. (Princess Diana has chronic back trouble, which some experts suggest might be due to the very high heels she often wears.) Also avoid thick platform shoes, which can throw body balance off and make it easy to turn your ankle and fall.

Try shoes with crepe soles or rubber heels to see if their shock-absorbing quality eliminates hip and back problems. For running or walking shoes, look for shoes with several layers of heel for adequate shock absorption.

Test different kinds of shoes and different heel heights to decide for yourself what makes your feet and back feel best. If you find a supershoe that fits just right and is comfortable, stay with that brand and style. If necessary, have your shoes custom-made.

The surgical team at the GCOC Institute almost all wear clogs with wooden soles, leather band on top, and low heels. The shoe forces you to walk with a slightly flexed knee so that the impact of the heel-strike goes partly to the knee and only slightly to the hip and back. You don't suffer as much shock to your spine. Even with long hours in the operating room standing on their feet, with the clogs the surgical team personnel no longer have sore backs. If you can't find clogs in a shoe store, you may be able to find them in a uniform or medical supply store. Try them around the house, learning to squeeze your foot forward with each step instead of walking heel first.

Whatever shoes you wear, you need to keep them in good repair—no rundown heels or other hazards to throw you off balance.

Go barefoot in the house, on grass, and in sand—it's good for your feet (but don't go barefoot on hard streets and sidewalks or where there is likelihood of infection).

Your Back and Your Bed

How to Choose the Best Bed for Your Back

You probably spend about one-third of your life in bed, so the bed you sleep in can be especially important to whether your back hurts or not.

You need a good mattress. Shop for one that will support your body weight evenly and efficiently and that will keep your spine in correct alignment. It should adjust to your body contours and be comfortable. Before you purchase a mattress, lie down on the samples in the store. See how they feel when you lie on them.

People with back problems should consult their physician about the kind of mattress best for their particular circumstances. For most people, a medium or firm mattress is best. Your mattress shouldn't be so soft that your body sags, or so firm that it might contribute to back and neck stiffness. If you awaken in the morning feeling refreshed and without any stiffness or backache, your mattress is probably fine.

If two people sleep in your bed, get a queen or king size. A double bed only allows the same width per person as a crib. When using a queen size, be sure there is a rigid center support on the bedframe to help distribute the weight of the mattress and prevent sagging. A king-size mattress should rest on two frames for better support. The frames can be locked together to prevent them from sliding around. Twin beds also can be placed together with a locking device in the center.

Turn and rotate a new mattress once a month during the first six months of use. After that, turn and rotate the mattress every three months.

Some people like the extra firmness of a bedboard. Some mattresses have a bedboard built right in, or you can simply slide a large piece of ¾-inch plywood (½-inch is too thin and will sag) under the mattress. Make sure the board extends completely from side to side and top to bottom.

If you are staying in a hotel and are used to a bedboard, ask the hotel to supply one. They are usually available.

Haven't got a bedboard? Take the mattress off the bed and put it on the floor. But be careful when you get up. It's sometimes possible to strain a muscle simply from standing suddenly from a low position.

What About Waterbeds?

Research on water, gel, and air mattresses has indicated that postoperative patients after back surgery are more comfortable on them, and long-term bedridden patients using them have fewer bedsores.

Some patients claim that waterbeds make their backs feel better than conventional mattresses; others don't like them. The only way to find out is to test one for yourself: rent one, sleep on one at a friend's house, or get a hotel room with one. Some companies will let customers try a waterbed for 30 days with a money-back guarantee if it doesn't suit.

Waterbeds have different degrees of firmness, depending on the amount of water in them. If the bed is too firm (too full), it may not provide the necessary conformity to the curves of the spine. If it is too soft, it may not give enough support.

Experiment with different amounts of water and find what's best for you.

Some mattresses have air chambers that eliminate water motion and lighten the weight of the unit. You might also consider a mattress filled with gel or air instead of water to see how they affect your back. Again, no matter what other people claim for their backs, you have to try it for yourself. What is good for one person is not necessarily best for another.

Best Sleeping Positions for Your Back

Use a pillow the right size for you—not so thick that it raises your head and neck and not so thin that your neck slopes downward. The goal is to have your neck follow your spine in a straight, level line. One of our patients found that taking half the stuffing from his pillow got rid of a backache he had had for four years.

If you read in bed, use pillows at the small of your back and behind your neck so that you can recline, not slump.

The best sleeping position is to lie on your side with hips and knees bent, arms in front of you, with your body partially curled. Some people also like to have a pillow between their knees in this position.

Others find it best for their backs to sleep on the stomach. Again, try it for yourself. In any event, everyone moves around during sleep so you won't stay in that position for the entire night.

Finding a comfortable sleeping position is especially difficult if you are pregnant. Lying on your side offers the least problems. Part of the problem for expectant mothers is that during the last weeks of pregnancy, a woman will lean backward to counterbalance the weight of the protruding abdomen, putting an excessive arch in the back. Because of this, tissues can be overstretched around the joints of the spine, causing backache. Because of the excessive arching, the pregnant woman should do the Pelvic Tilt exercises that tend to flatten the back, but not extension exercises such as the tired horse that arch the back even further.

How Not to Have a Tired Back when You Are Bedridden

1. Place a pillow under the knees.
2. Place a box or two pillows at the foot of the bed to rest the feet against and to raise the sheets or blankets off the feet.
3. Try a bedboard that is split into three sections. It makes it possible to support the back and raise the knees like a hospital bed. Split bedboards with supports can be bought in most hospital supply stores or can be improvised with plywood.
4. To keep from getting stiff muscles and to prevent bedsores, get into a new position frequently. (If you are to be in bed for a very long time, this would be the time to consider getting a water or gel mattress. Insurance often will pay for purchase or rental.)
5. To help keep muscles from getting very weak, (a) contract the muscles of your legs and buttocks and hold; (b) pull your abdomen in as flat as you can and push your shoulders back; (c) raise your legs, one at a time. Do as many times a day as you can.
6. As soon as you are allowed to be ambulatory, get out of bed as often as you can to sit in a chair or take short walks.

How to Get Out of Bed

Getting out of bed in the morning can be a peak injury time. Your muscles may still be stiff, your ligaments tight, and your mind sleepy. Wait a few minutes after waking up before you get out of bed, stretch and relax, and then get up. Some people find it helpful to do their back exercises while they are lying there thinking about the coming day.

Get out of bed slowly. Roll to your side, slip your feet over the edge of the bed, use your arms to push your trunk up, sit for a moment, then stand up slowly. This slow way of getting up is also good for people who have postural hypotension (getting dizzy from a drop in blood pressure when they stand up too quickly).

What to Do for Your Back when You Walk

Most back pain sufferers should start their walking program with a ½ mile the first day or two, then gradually build up to the longer distances. The best of the patients of GCOC are up to 5 miles a day.

The problem is that the way cities are being built and automobiles being used today, most of us don't walk anymore. But you need to walk. Start out with a walk around your neighborhood today; then find a friend to walk with you on a regular basis to help keep you motivated.

Watch your posture when you walk. Stand tall, head up, shoulders back, gut in. Don't waddle; keep your steps even and in a straight line.

The way to walk is for men to take long steps and women to take smaller steps. This is because with a woman's anatomy, the pelvis is larger and tilts at an angle, so that if a woman takes long steps, it tilts the pelvis too much, putting added pressure on the sacroiliac joint and causing rotation of the spine. Indeed, because a woman has more movement in her skeleton throughout life when walking, she has more potential for degenerative changes in the spine. (Pregnancy makes it even more accented, since it causes even more widening and tilting of the pelvis.)

Men usually have a flat narrower pelvis so that their legs can go straighter in longer steps.

What to Do for Your Back when You Drive

The way you sit when you drive can bring on back problems. Just like sitting in a chair, remember not to slump. Look for cars with firm, but not hard, seats and those with extra lumbar support. Many foreign and American cars now have ergonomically designed seats that are adjustable to give maximum support to the small of the back. Use a backrest if needed, or put a pillow behind your back. Be wary of low sports cars that are difficult to get in and out of. Also check that any car you buy has an adequate headrest to prevent injury if you are rear-ended.

Be sure seats are far enough forward so that you don't have to stretch your legs to reach the pedals or your arms to reach the wheel.

Keep your head and shoulders erect. If you lean forward, you'll develop pains in your neck and back. Avoid tensing your muscles. Be alert but relaxed enough to keep muscles from cramping.

Change your position in whatever way you can; have a co-driver when possible on long trips, even if the other person only drives for short periods. It gives you a chance to change position, perhaps to stretch out on the back seat.

Carry food and drink with you, especially protein foods to give you long-lasting energy.

When lifting a suitcase or tire in or out of a trunk, place a foot into the trunk or on the bumper.

The Better Back Auto Break

One factor that aggravates back problems more than anything else is long periods of uninterrupted sitting, whether you are the passenger or the driver. It's not only the sitting in one position that affects you, but also the vibration of the car that causes muscle fatigue. Many highways have undulations at an average of every 15 feet, causing a phenomenon called the California highway hop. Not good for the back.

Help your fatigue, and your back, by making a stop every hour or two. Walk around. Do the following exercises.

1. Grasp your left wrist with your right hand and your right wrist with your left hand. Raise your arms to shoulder height. Attempt to pull your arms apart for a count of 6. Repeat 3 times.
2. Put your right hand against the side of your head and push your head against it. Put your left hand against the side of your head and push against it. Lock fingers behind your head and push your head back against them. Do each slowly 3 times.
3. Place your right fist in the palm of your left hand, arms shoulder high. Press as hard as you can, resisting with the left hand for a count of 6. Do 3 times. Repeat with the other hand.
4. Put your right hand on your right shoulder, your left hand on your left shoulder. Rotate your elbows forward, up, then back, making small circles. Do 5 times. Then do it with your arms outstretched, doing windmills.
5. Stand at the side of the car with one hand on the car for support. Keep your back straight and do deep knee bends, squatting down to the ground and up. Do 3 times slowly.
6. Put one foot up on the side or trunk of the car and stretch gently toward the car in a sort of fencer's thrust. Do 5 times. Switch to the other leg.
7. Have a snack and a drink of water, take a little walk again, and get back in the car refreshed.

How to Lift and Carry Without Straining Your Back

Many back problems could be avoided if people understood

75

good body mechanics, and learned how to lift and do other work. If the subject were taught in grade and high school, millions of dollars would be saved in medical bills later.

Here are things to remember:

1. Never lean over from the waist with legs straight to pick something up, even a feather. One woman who came to the Institute had bent down to pick up a baby stroller and stressed her back so badly the pain took her to the emergency room the next morning and she had to be flat on her back in bed and in traction for a week.

2. Never let your back carry the exertion or load. Whether you are picking up a box, a baby, or a handkerchief, always bend your knees when lifting. Place your feet close to the object, with your feet about 8 to 12 inches apart; keep your back upright, and bend at the knees to a squat position; lift slowly and smoothly, using the leg muscles.

3. Do not strain the neck muscles.

4. Hold objects close to your body. A light weight held at arm's length produces more stress on the spine than does a heavier weight held close to the body.

5. If you are doing heavy lifting, bend backward several times before and after lifting.

6. Don't wear high heels when lifting; it increases the stress.

7. Don't lean over a piece of furniture to lift a stuck window.

8. Avoid lifting anything heavy over your head.

9. Do not twist while holding a heavy object.

10. Don't lift if your footing is insecure; a slip or twist can wrench your back. If carrying for a distance, make sure your pathway is clear.

11. If a load is too heavy, *do not lift it!* Wait for someone to help you.

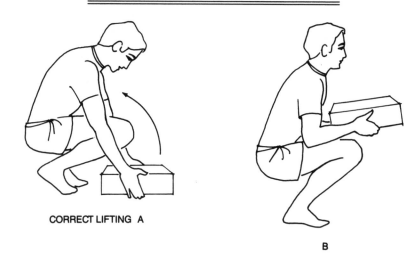

CORRECT LIFTING A

B

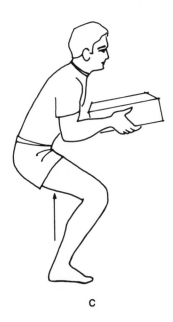

C

12. Don't keep trying to lift an object if you feel any discomfort in your back. If you have back trouble, don't even try to lift heavy objects. Let someone else do it.

One patient who came to the Institute had such a weak back that the slightest lifting caused her pain. She was even afraid to pick up her new infant daughter. However, when she followed the advice on lifting, she was able to lift her baby again.

Pushing and Pulling

1. Never try to move a heavy piece of furniture by yourself. Get one or two people to help you, and work together as a team, first determining the direction you will both move, then lifting simultaneously so that both people share the weight equally.
2. To push, place hands on object, bend knees so arms are level with the object. Walk, pushing the object in front of you.
3. To pull, grasp the object, bend your knees so your arms are level with the object, and walk backward pulling with your entire body weight rather than just with your arms or back.
4. Use a wheelbarrow, dolly, or other mechanical aid whenever possible.
5. If you have a choice, it is better to push than to pull.

How to Have Good Sex With a Bad Back

A bad back almost never need keep you from having sex. In fact, sex can help your back. It can provide exercise, relieve tension, give a sense of well-being, and actually help ease pain. Many arthritis patients say they achieve six to eight hours of relief from pain after sexual activity.

(However, sometimes a person may be in such pain that it

inhibits sexual desire, or there may be lessening of sexual desire as a side effect of medications for back pain, such as corticosteroids. If this happens, the doctor may be able to lower the dosage or substitute another medication.)

Six Rules for Success

1. If you are having a severe attack of back pain, it will be safer for you not to have sex until a day after the attack is over, when sex should be no problem.
2. If you have had back pain, try sexual activities gradually. Judge by where you are in the exercise program. The farther advanced you are in your back-strengthening exercises, the more adventurous you may be with your sexual activities.
3. Engage in sex when you are well rested rather than when you—and your back—are fatigued. A hot bath or gentle massage can be a body-relaxing and muscle-limbering prelude.
4. Do not use acrobatic positions that could put a strain on your back. Avoid violent or sudden jarring or twisting movements, and concentrate instead on smooth, slow, sensuous movements.
5. Keep the back as straight as possible or only slightly arched—nearly any position is safe as long as you avoid those that put your back in a severe swayback position that arches the back greatly.
6. If back pain occurs, stop immediately, wait for the pain to subside, then begin again slowly in a different position. If the pain is severe, then do not continue, but consult with your doctor for his or her recommendations.

The Best Sex Positions for the Person with a Bad Back

The least stressful position for either the man or the woman with a bad back is lying on the back with the knees slightly bent, flattening the lower back against the mattress. Think back to your exercises: if you combine the Flat Back Pelvic Tilt exercise with the Pelvic Raise exercise, you can have very effective stimulation and not only protect the back, but even strengthen it by the exercise. The exercise is most beneficial (and the stimulation very effective) if movements are done very, very slowly. The partner with the bad back can also place a pillow under the buttocks for extra support and to help keep the back from arching too much.

The "spoon" position is also excellent when one or both partners has a bad back: the woman lies on her side with knees bent, the man lying behind her, curling about her and penetrating from behind. A variation of this position is for the woman to put a pillow between her knees to keep the top leg from twisting and overstretching the muscles of the hip and back.

In all these positions, the sexual push-pulling, if done gently and properly, is excellent therapy for building a stronger back. Keep up the back exercise program. As your back feels stronger and better, you should be able to perform sexually with even more freedom.

A Sex Stretch

If you have hip or back pain during or after sexual inter-course, or if you have trouble stretching your legs wide, this exercise may be of help:

Stand in front of a table or bench that is about as high as your hips. Turn the foot (of the leg you are standing on) strongly in. Stretch the other leg straight out and rest your heel on the table. Bend forward from the hip, reaching toward your outstretched foot with both hands, and very gently keep stretching, trying to reach farther toward your foot each time. Reach 10 to 20 times; then switch to the other leg and reach 10 to 20 times.

Other Posture and Back Improvers

1. Don't sit with one foot up under you.
2. Don't always stand with your weight on one foot.
3. Put a foot up on a 5- or 6-inch-high stool or step if you have to stand for a long time. (Perhaps it's no coincidence that bars have foot railings. Putting one foot up on the rail is relaxing because it takes the strain off your back. You can stay longer—and drink more!)
4. Don't use heavy shoulder bags routinely; when you do use a shoulder bag, alternate from one shoulder to the other. When you carry things, divide them into two equal loads, one shopping bag or suitcase for each arm.
5. Don't hold the phone by hunching one shoulder up and cocking your head.
6. Don't slouch, even if you think it's cool or you are embarrassed at being extra tall.
7. When you walk down the street, occasionally glance at your reflection in a store window. If you see your head jutting forward or your body slouched, realign your body.
8. Keep thinking about how the way you carry your body reflects the way you feel about yourself. Feel proud and stand tall.

CHAPTER SIX

How to Protect Your Back at Work

Of course, jobs that involve much bending and twisting, or lifting heavy objects, are bad for your back, but so are jobs that involve long periods of sitting or standing in one place. Dentists and surgeons often suffer from back pain because they stand all day, secretaries because they sit all day, and truck drivers because they not only sit for long periods with constant vibration of the truck, but they also often lift and strain with heavy deliveries.

However, no matter what your occupation, you can find things to do to help your back and keep it in better shape. Check this list for tips that can help you.

If you are a student, don't always carry heavy piles of books on one hip. Switch sides. Try not to slouch at your desk, even though the desk is out of proportion and uncomfortable. Tell your parents or your doctor if you notice that your spine is slightly curved to the side instead of straight.

If you are a traveling salesman, don't always carry your briefcase on one side. Watch your driving posture. Take exercise breaks during long drives. Learn to relax between customer calls.

If you are a waiter or waitress, walk with a springy gait instead of a jarring one, to lessen shock to the spine. Wear well-fitting shoes with broad rubber soles and heels. Do not stand with your knees pushed back and the back excessively curved, which so many waiters do when standing at their stations. Lift and lower heavy trays with a gradual, fluid motion, not suddenly or jerkily.

If you are a nurse, the biggest danger to your back is lifting patients. Never try to lift a patient while you are bent over. Get help whenever possible. When you have to lift, protect yourself by lifting with your hip and leg muscles, not with back muscles.

If you are a secretary, make sure the typewriter isn't too far away from you when you type. If you get shoulder, neck, or back pains, it can be from frequent reaching behind you at an awkward angle. Try rearranging your desk and files to keep from reaching in strained positions. When placing things in a bottom file drawer, squat rather than bend over.

If you are a carpenter, try to avoid spending a long time using one tool in one repetitive motion. Be careful lifting doors, windows, or other heavy things when you can't get proper leverage—get someone to help you. Try to avoid pounding nails overhead while perched on top of a ladder. Try to get in a less awkward position.

When you are ironing, if your back gets tired, get away from the ironing board for a while and stretch out on your back, or do a job that doesn't use the same arm.

If you are cleaning the bathtub, clean it before you get out. If you're cleaning it from the outside, kneel and use a long-handled brush so you don't have to bend your back.

If you work overhead, reaching up can put a strain on the back and shoulder muscles. Put your arms down as frequently as you can. If you wear bifocals and have neck pains, it could be that you're straining your neck and thrusting your head forward to see overhead through the bifocals. If you will be working at this job for quite some time, consult your optometrist or ophthalmologist about the possibility of having glasses made with the correct focus for that particular job.

If you are shoveling snow or digging a garden, consider letting someone else do it, such as a neighborhood teenager who would like to make a few dollars. If you do it yourself, do it slowly and rhythmically, holding the shovel as close to the body as possible. As you shovel, bend your knees, not your waist, to take some strain off your back. Turn the body by shifting the feet rather than twisting the trunk. When you shovel, lighten the strain by sliding one hand down the shaft and using it as a fulcrum, while you push the end of the handle down with the other hand. When you have a very heavy shovelful, bend one knee and brace the handle against the thigh as a fulcrum.

When you weed a garden, kneel or sit instead of bending over. Remember when you do any job with prolonged forward bending and stooping you should stand up at regular intervals and bend backward several times—before pain starts.

If you lay floors or carpets, your problem is the constant bent-over position. Change your position as frequently as you can. Try to relax neck and shoulder muscles while you are working instead of keeping them tensely scrunched up. If you get the chance, occasionally lie down on your back on that beautiful new carpet, flattening your back to the floor for a few minutes.

If you are a salesperson, when you are between customers, guard against slumping into bad posture habits. Stand relaxed and, to stimulate circulation, make small repeated contractions of the muscles in your abdomen, feet, and legs.

If you are a musician or an orchestra leader, you probably remain in one position for long stretches of time, repeating the same movements, using the same muscles. Drummers, for example, tend to develop pains in the shoulders; organists get lower back pain and pains in the leg muscles. Try to put whatever muscles are getting sore and cramped through a wide range of motions between sets. Raise your arms above your head and do windmill circles; then do shoulder shrugs. Elevate your feet and legs if you have been sitting in a cramped position.

If you are a truck driver, use a backrest with support for the small of your back, and on long trips take frequent breaks for food and exercise. Even helping load and unload the truck helps to counteract the inactivity from sitting long periods. If you drive a truck with a hard seat or poor springs, use a thick sponge-rubber cushion to avoid pain of the tailbone.

If you operate foot pedals, you may develop pain in the lower back if you reach for pedals with one foot. Mail handlers who habitually kick mail sacks with one foot may develop the same trouble. Use both feet equally if you can, and bend your extended leg occasionally. Stand up when the leg is fatigued and walk about or swing the leg back and forth and shake it.

When you vacuum, stand straight rather than stooping over. Don't twist.

When you hoe, rake, mop, or sweep, stand sideways with your feet fairly wide apart and use the implement in a left-to-right motion instead of forward and back in front of you, which puts constant tension on the back and shoulder muscles. Don't bend over.

If you are a dentist, sit on a stool when you can. Adjust the patient's chair and your work tables to proper heights for you, so you do not have to hunch and bend over so much. Change your position during operative procedures as much as you can. Avoid working with your weight on one leg.

If you stand a lot on any job, wear the best-fitting shoes you can find. Consider wearing support stockings. Try to put one foot up on something whenever possible.

If you work at a table or sink, make sure that the work surface height is not too high and that the lighting is not poor, making you strain your neck and back. Table height should be about 2 inches below your elbows. (To measure, keep your arms at your side and bend your elbows to 90 degrees.) For activities that require fine detail, use a work surface that is slightly higher. You should avoid working bent over or with your head bent forward or sideways.

If you are a police officer, take care not to get a sore heel from walking so much. (If you get a sore heel, put a rubber pad with a hole in it in your shoe where your heel hurts, which will take the weight off the painful area, or see a podiatrist.) Do not let a painful foot go untreated because you may develop an abnormal way of walking that can cause leg and back problems.

If you are in the military, your feet and consequently your back may often give you trouble. Soldiers often get stress fractures in their feet during long marches. Make sure that you have shoes that fit, and if marching gives you problems, check with a therapist on muscle-strengthening exercises for the feet and legs that will help prevent fractures.

If you fly long distances, backache is often produced because of the muscle fatigue that occurs when one sits inactively in one position for such a long time. Do each of the following exercises 5 or 6 times in your seat.

1. Tighten and relax the muscles of the left thigh, then the right thigh.
2. Squeeze the muscles of the buttocks together; hold and relax.
3. Try to tighten and relax the muscles of the back.
4. Contract the muscles of your shoulders; then relax them.
5. Flatten the back of the neck against the seat back.
6. Stretch upward, lifting the neck with chin in; then press

elbows against the seat back until your body is forced forward from the seat back; then relax.

7. Put both arms on the arm rests. Try to bring the shoulder blades together in the back. Now press both elbows down to act as levers to lift the body, and relax.

8. Press the right hand on the left knee and try to lift the knee. Press hard so you cannot lift it. Repeat with the opposite hand and knee.

Don't sit in the seat for too long a time. Get up and walk around several times during the flight. If the plane stops en route, get off and walk around. (But don't miss your plane!)

CHAPTER SEVEN

How to Protect Your Back in Sports

Bill was in terrible shape because of lack of exercise, and he was overweight. He vowed to improve, lost 30 pounds, then got out his old tennis shoes and started jogging around the neighborhood. The next day he couldn't walk because of the severe back pain.

Bill's story is typical. Many people who are in poor shape because they have not exercised for years start up with some sport for exercise with the best of intentions—but they begin too strenuously, don't learn the proper precautions to protect themselves from damage, or choose a sport that is damaging instead of beneficial.

This is why our program begins with gradual back exercises plus a walking program. The combination strengthens your muscles and builds up your general condition gradually. Only after several weeks of conditioning should you, if you wish, begin a more strenuous sport.

Even if you begin a more strenuous sport, we recommend— as do other back experts—that you continue walking and/or swimming to continue building your back strength and your general condition. Walking and swimming will give you continued conditioning along with and in between the times you engage in other sports.

Walking and swimming will also give you a high aerobic fitness benefit for your heart and lungs and will help trim away fat. One of these activities should be done at least three times a week for maximum benefit.

Remember the importance of cross-training. The American College of Sports Medicine is revising its fitness guidelines, recommending that in addition to aerobic exercise, adults of all ages should also do strength training. The cross-training allows you to develop a strong, flexible well-proportioned body in addition to a healthy heart and lungs. We've built that concept into our Better Back exercise program (Chapter 4), and you also should think of it when you choose the sports you want to participate in.

As in any exercise activity, you need to review with your doctor what is best for you and your back before beginning a sport. If your doctor approves, and if the sport makes you feel good, do it and enjoy it. If it makes your back hurt, discontinue it.

Of course, don't forget to check your cardiovascular fitness too. A rule of thumb: After exercise, your heart rate should take no longer than 5 minutes to return to resting levels.

Ten Basic Rules for Any Sport if You Have a Weak Back

1. Get your doctor's approval before starting.
2. Begin working at the sport gradually, and build up time and endurance in gradual stages.
3. If any particular sport or movement produces pain, avoid it.
4. Spend a few minutes walking or doing warm-up exercises appropriate to the sport before each session.

5. Avoid sudden, awkward, jarring moves. A quick shift off balance can throw even a healthy back askew.
6. Low-impact exercise is better than exercise that compresses the discs or twists the back.
7. Choose a sport that releases tension, not one that adds to it.
8. Obtain professional instruction to be sure that you are using proper nonstressing techniques.
9. If you are a weekend exerciser only, be sure to do the walking we recommend or other exercising during the week to avoid being out of shape.
10. Remember that children can develop back damage too. Never tell your children to "train through pain."

Hazardous Sports If You Have a Bad Back

You should avoid sports that involve rough physical contact, or those in which there is twisting or severe arching of the back, or those where there is danger of sudden impact or jarring.

Football, for example, is an extremely dangerous sport for the head, neck, and spine. One bad tackle or head butt could mean a shock to the spine that could cause immediate back problems, or could result in serious trouble later in life. The biggest danger is the impact to the head in blocking and tackling. In one study, 32 percent of players x-rayed were found to have fractures, disc problems, and limited motion—just from playing football in high school. The Arthritis Foundation warns that 50 to 80 percent of high school and college football players are eventually injured and that many, because of the injuries, will have serious joint pain later in life.

Many other sports are dangerous too. A study just published in Sweden shows that the severe twists and landings performed by top gymnasts is causing damage to their spines. Two dozen gymnasts, aged 18 to 29, on the Swedish national gymnastic team were studied and compared to nongymnasts. "The number of degenerated discs among the gymnasts was comparable to what you expect to see in 65-year-old men," according to Dr. Richard Nymann at the University Hospital in Uppsala, Sweden. Many had misaligned vertebrae and bulging discs and most had back pain.

If you have a bad back, avoid all of the following: basketball, board diving, bowling, football, gymnastics, handball, high-jumping, hurdles, ice hockey, pole vaulting, sledding, tobogganing, snowmobiling, soccer, trampoline, volleyball, and wrestling.

What About Jogging?

If you have a healthy back, jogging and running are excellent conditioners. If you have a back problem, there could be trouble.

If you want to run, check with your doctor about your particular condition, and if you are given the go-ahead, get proper training so that you will have the proper form.

Then get off on the right foot by getting into condition first. Build up slowly and easily. Most runners find that after completing our exercise program their muscles don't tire as easily and they seem to have more power in their stride as they run.

Under no circumstances should you run on concrete or asphalt, which are punishing to bone and joints. Instead, run on soft surfaces like park fields and athletic trails. Wear shoes with thick rubber soles and arch supports and soft, well-fitting socks to help cushion jarring to the spine. Once you find a comfortable shoe that doesn't produce injuries, stick to it, since many running injuries occur when runners switch from one brand of shoe to another. When you get a new pair of shoes, start breaking them in before the old ones fall apart so that the body will adapt to the new shoes.

When you run, stay loose—don't waste energy gritting your teeth or tensing your muscles. Run in an upright position—don't lean. Keep your buttocks tucked in—don't run with a swayback. Don't look at your feet. To limit the jarring on your spine, make your gait low and smooth—don't bounce.

Don't run downhill; it puts excessive strain on the knees and back. Walk when you have to go downhill. If you run on sand, run near the water where the sand if firmer; it places less stress on the back.

If you become unusually tired or uncomfortable, slow down, walk, or stop.

Tennis

Tennis is a sport that can be beneficial to your fitness if done properly, but it can cause severe backache when done wrong. Poor strokes, such as hitting the ball too late, cause the most injuries. If you want to play tennis, take lessons from a pro.

Get in condition with our walking program and back exercises before you start playing. When you do start, gradually build up the intensity and length of time you play. Every time you play, warm up with some limbering exercises before you go on the court. On the first few days, take a hot shower or hot tub soak after the workout to prevent stiffness and discomfort. If you are a weekend player, keep in condition between games.

If your back starts to bother you, stay off hard-surface courts and play only on clay or grass.

Walking and Hiking

As we have been saying all along, walking and hiking are

wonderful for the person with a bad back. That's why walking is so much a part of our exercise program. However, watch out for "rucksack palsy" from hiking with a heavy load on your back. The symptoms include pain, numbness, and weakness in the back, shoulders, and arms because of pressure of the backpack on nerves and blood vessels. You can avoid it by using a backpack with thick foam-rubber cushioning under the shoulder straps and metal supports to distribute the load onto hips. There should be as little pressure on the shoulders as possible. At the first sign of discomfort, remove and lighten pack. If you have back trouble, don't carry a backpack at all.

Wear comfortable shoes when you walk or hike. Things to look for are: a well-cushioned heel for shock absorption, a flexible forefoot, and a well-fitting toe box.

Swimming

Remember from our chapter on pool exercises that the back-stroke is the best back-strengthening swimming stroke. The crawl and sidestroke are also good. If the exercises that arched your back were helpful to you, then the breast- or butterfly stroke might be helpful also, but if arching exercises made your back feel worse, then don't do the breaststroke or butterfly. In fact, competitive swimmers when training often get what orthopedic specialists call "butterfly back syndrome" because of the repetitive extension and flexion that occurs with this stroke, especially with racing starts and turns.

No matter what strokes you use, work up to swimming distances gradually. If you have a bad back, don't dive off the board.

Holding on to the side of the pool and kicking is a good hip exercise.

If you are having an attack of back pain, avoid swimming in

water below 70 degrees and take a hot shower after swimming to avoid being chilled.

Golf

If you choose golf for your sport, be sure when you play not to lean backward at the completion of the swing trying to watch the ball. Also be careful to squat or bend at the hips and knees when you place or retrieve the golf ball. Keep your play relaxed and focus on keeping your body in alignment and balance.

Limit the hours you play until you have tested the effect of the game on your back.

Bicycling

How you ride your bike can affect your back. A bicycle should fit the rider: pick the right-size frame, put the seat at the proper height, and adjust the length and height of the handlebars and the distance of the seat so that it is comfortable for you. Choose a bicycle with handlebars that help you keep your back straight instead of hunched over. Use a padded seat and don't ride over bumpy surfaces that jar your back. Don't ride with a backpack. At the times when your back is bothering you, don't ride a bike at all.

Dancing

Done properly, dancing can help extend the spine, improve posture, increase flexibility, and increase coordination. It helps use up calories and keeps you trim, and sometimes is even aerobic. However, the person preventing back problems should avoid the twist, the duck walk, splits, and other back-stressing maneuvers.

The proper body alignment when dancing is to pull the

stomach in and up, the derriere under, and the shoulders back. Stand tall and relaxed. Move mainly on the front half of your feet or even flat-footed, but not high on your toes.

Horseback Riding

If you have a healthy back, horseback riding can be good exercise. However, riding is often bad for low back pain sufferers and those with disc problems. Ride with your back straight or slightly curved, but not with an exaggerated curve in it. Take lessons for proper form.

If you have a bad back, you should check with your doctor before riding, and test the effect for yourself, since different people seem to react in different ways.

Check saddle, stirrups, and bridle carefully and frequently.

If You Work Out in a Gym

Working out on exercise equipment is fine, but you must be very careful of what you use and what you do, never straining or overworking your back. Before you jump in and start working out, have a fitness analysis done by a physical therapist or other fitness expert at the gym who will then give you a schedule of which exercises are best for you and how often you should do them as you gradually work up to more strength. This is what we do at the Institute.

If you are like the typical back pain sufferer, you probably will need to work with the types of equipment that strengthen your back extensor muscles and abdominal muscles and those that gently stretch your hamstrings.

An excellent machine for the back is the NordicTrack, which mimics the workout of cross-country skiing. It provides overall strengthening of the neck, shoulders, and upper and lower back. The lower back, especially, is strengthened by the resistance and the opposing actions of the leg and arm motions. In addition, because you are standing, this is a weight-bearing exercise, good for strengthening bones and helping to prevent osteoporosis. It is also excellent for total-body and cardiovascular fitness, particularly because it exercises the upper and lower body simultaneously.

Some fitness centers may also have the new Lumbar Extension Machine, which was recently designed by Arthur Jones, developer of Nautilus; at present, however, the equipment is available mostly in a few doctors' offices. It particularly works the lumbar extensor muscles on each side of the spine in the lower back. We will tell you more about it in Chapter 11, when we discuss treatments.

When you exercise, warm up for a while on a treadmill or stationary bicycle or by using the NordicTrack slowly and easily.

When you start out on any fitness equipment, work at the slowest speed and don't worry too much about technique. At the first session, do some stretching first, use the machine for a minute or two, then dismount and walk around to make sure there is no increased back pain, then get back on for another minute to two. This is enough time for the first session. Gradually increase the time until you get up to what is recommended for you. Do *not* work too long at your first sessions (sometimes it feels so good, you are tempted, but you will be sorry later), and as with any exercise, if pain becomes worse, discontinue the exercise and consult your physician.

Back patients, in general, are better off not using weights unless they work regularly with a good instructor. Otherwise, you could worsen your back problem instead of helping it. If you do use weight machines, use those that let you rest your back against a support. Be sure that you keep your back straight; don't arch it or round it as you lift.

How to Keep Your Child from Being Injured in Sports

Children should be encouraged to take up sports they can enjoy all their lives, such as tennis and swimming, not just team sports.

Avoid dangerous sports such as football and intense competition for your child in any sport, especially if it makes the child push himself or herself beyond his or her limits. Anyone who plays under tension or overexerts himself is more vulnerable to injury.

Give your child professional instruction when possible so that self-confidence and skills can be developed from the beginning and the clumsiness that often leads to injury avoided.

Most people don't think of children as having back problems, but they do get them. If your child complains of an aching back don't brush it off—believe the complaint. Never, never tell a child to continue a sport if he is in pain. With growing bones and young cartilage, a child can easily stress himself and cause permanent damage. This is especially important in light of new research that shows that many children have hidden structural defects of the spine, even disc degeneration, that appears to be inherited. Not all spines are created equal, and what one child may be able to do, another cannot do without damage. In fact, that's true of adults, too.

For children or adults, if there is a predisposition to back problems, it is doubly important to build strength in the back.

CHAPTER EIGHT

How to Fight Tensions That Can Tighten Your Back

Our daily lives sometimes seem filled with stressful events. The usual result—adrenalin levels go up, blood pressure goes up, the heart beats faster, muscles tense. With the tension, many of us contract the muscles of the back, shoulders, or neck, holding them stiff and tense in one position. By the end of the day, we may have a headache, fatigue, and a stiff neck, or our back may hurt so much we could cry.

Sometimes the connection between tension and backache is obvious. The tension connection comes because you have been hunched over the typewriter or drawing board all day, frantically trying to make a deadline you know is impossible, or you have been grimly shoveling snow or clutching a phone all afternoon with neck bent sideways and shoulder bunched up. In these cases, you know why you have a backache.

At other times the tension connection is more subtle. A long-term problem may be keeping you tense without your realizing it, causing fatigue and backache. One patient said that at the end of almost every workday his neck felt as if someone was tightening a noose around it. His job was causing him tremendous stress. It was literally a pain in the neck. Often the pain traveled from his neck to his shoulders and back. Sometimes his muscles were so tight and sore that he would have difficulty driving his car because he couldn't turn his head to see to the side of the car. After he had training in stress reduction, his neck and his back pain gradually left him.

Sometimes backache is tied into depression. A depressed person frequently walks and sits in a slumped position, which can cause backache. Thus it becomes a vicious cycle—you become more depressed because of the pain, which results in even less movement and worse posture, which causes more muscle contraction and more pain.

Sometimes the problems can be made even worse. Whether your back is tense from a bad day, the emotional strain from a long-term problem, or depression, your muscles are tight and braced. Then even a minor physical twist or strain can trigger a painful spasm, compounding the problem.

It can also work the other way around. First, you have a back problem; then you add emotional tension to that. Research shows that people with chronic back problems often have severe flareups and attacks during or immediately after periods of great tension. The first triggering episode of back trouble may be physical straining, lifting, or falling, but after that, the attacks of pain are often correlated with periods of unhappiness and tension or other emotional upset.

There is one unique characteristic that the back patients who react to tension seem to have in common. They often are found to contract more muscles for longer times when trying to accomplish something—often unnecessarily. For example, when asked to squeeze a doctor's fingers as hard as possible, such a patient may grit his teeth, hunch up both shoulders, raise his shoulders, and even after the test, exhibit tense muscles.

The Key to the Tension/Muscle Connection

The truth is that you don't have to hurt your back for your back to hurt. This does not mean that your back pain is all in your head, but it does mean that you may have to work to cope better with the stress that may be in your life.

The key is usually a combination of strengthening the muscles through exercise, plus learning to relax, mentally and physically.

Sometimes part of the key is simply knowing that tension or anger can be the cause of a back episode. Then you can learn to recognize when you are angry or tense and to let tensed muscles relax.

How to Check Yourself for Clues to Hidden Tension

Could unrecognized tension be causing you to have backache? Most of us are unaware of when stress is getting to us and we are building up tension. Perhaps you are more tense then you realize.

There are clues to tension you can learn to recognize. For example, check yourself on whether you have anxiety and tension right now. Is your jaw clenched? Are you biting your teeth together? Are the muscles in your back tight?

You can cut down on your tension-muscle connection by stopping periodically throughout the day—whenever you think you might be under stress, suffering from anxiety, or hurrying—and checking yourself for some of these clues to hidden tension:

Tight neck or jaw muscles

Tight shoulders or back

Gritting or grinding teeth

Tight, strained voice

Tightly curled toes or fingers

Irritability, overreacting to small things

Frowning

Smoking intensely

When you feel these signs coming on, take several deep breaths and consciously relax. The sooner you can do it, the better, before your muscles start to tighten. You don't *have* to grip the phone grimly when you talk, or pound your feet when you walk, or rush headlong through your work. Slow your talk, slow your walk, relax the fingers holding a pencil or telephone, and ease your mind and body into a relaxed approach to whatever you are doing. One of the GCOC patients bothered a lot by tension says that when she feels tense or depressed, she plays waltzes, or imagines them, to change her mood. Another patient uses the technique of smiling at the first sign of tension; another imagines standing under a waterfall to wash the tension away so that she can get to the problem without wasted energy.

Even when there is no way to eliminate the stress or crisis, you can learn to stop in the middle of a situation and mentally check for tight muscles and other signs of tension. The very act of checking often helps keep you from being tense.

You Can Save Your Back Later by Reducing Tensions Now

One of the important recent insights from psychology is that it isn't hard work that causes unhealthy stress; it is the feeling of being in a situation over which we have no control, one that we can't see how to handle. It's the frustration, anxiety, and tension of being unable to do something about a situation that needs changing, for example, the family or job problem that you have no control over and see no way to fix.

The other important insight that psychologists have learned is that is isn't the stressful situation itself that usually causes a problem, it's our attitude and reaction toward the situation. If you meet minor happenings as though they were major crises, you are more likely to experience the unhealthy effects of stress. How much a burned dinner, milk spilled, a flat tire, a bill unpaid, a client lost, a child crying affect you depends on the way you react to them.

You can start to reduce tension by simply learning to have a less frenzied, anxious reaction to life. One patient, when he gets tense, sits in a rocking chair and rocks slowly until he calms down. Another gets out of the house and takes a long walk. Another, when she finds herself pounding along, snapping at everybody and everything, hangs limp for a few moments, then very purposefully slows her walk and breathes more deeply.

Changing a Stressful Lifestyle

Here are some other techniques to help you reduce tension and cope with stress. They are not easy to carry out, but the more you aim for them, the better off you'll be, and not just in terms of back pain.

- Organize your day for the things you really want or need to do, so you are not always struggling against time. Keep lists of things to do. Carry a notebook for jotting down notes. At night check your calendar for engagements and plan your coming day.
- Have goals. Think about what you really want from life. List specific goals for the next few months and for the future. It will help you use your time toward your real goals rather than toward busy-busy trivia.
- Learn to concentrate on a task when you do it. Don't let your mind wander to other problems while you're taking

care of the current one. Try to eliminate distracting noises and conflicting activities.

- Use small bits of time. Carry a book to read, a letter to write, or other project to do during any waiting or commuting time. Cut down on TV time and, instead, use an hour in the evening for a hobby or to get a small job done.
- Try to make your work something you really like. Research has shown that there is a correlation between tension and job satisfaction. Take a look at your job. What could you do to make it better? If you feel inadequate, find out about some courses or books to improve your skills, or talk to your boss about switching to another job you think will fit you better.
- Do you often get angry? Do you always try to edge out the other person on the highway or get mad when you discuss things? Sometimes just stepping back and listening to yourself will help you recognize and stop destructive angry feelings.
- If boredom or loneliness is your problem, think about ways to bring some laughter and positive energies into your life. Try to make some new friends who are positive and have a sense of humor, volunteer to help solve a problem in your area, choose to go to a funny movie, watch a funny television show, read a funny book.
- If you are tense or angry, it can help to do something physical. Relax by gardening or cleaning out a closet. Take a walk, hit a ball, go to a dance, go for a swim. Exercise reduces tension. (Our exercise program will give you tension-relieving effects as well as back-strengthening.)

Instant Relief Techniques to Help Your Tension and Your Back

Head roll. Drop your chin to your chest. Rotate your head to the right and turn your chin to your shoulder. Circle your head slightly back and around and over your left shoulder to make a complete revolution. Repeat in the opposite direction.

Head tilt. Keep shoulders down. Tilt the left ear to the left shoulder several times. Tilt the right ear to the right shoulder several times.

The rag doll. Stand with your legs apart and bend at the waist. Keep your knees slightly bent. Shake your arms and hands loosely. Shrug your shoulders. Let your head hang, and sway from side to side.

Head lift. Curl your fingers around the sides of your neck, fingers meeting in back. Lift straight upward and forward as though you were trying to lift your head off your shoulders. Turn your head slightly from right to left while you continue lifting.

The sighing breath. Inhale deeply through the nostrils; then with lips puckered (as if cooling soup), exhale very slowly through the mouth for as long as you can. Concentrate on the long sighing sound and feel the tension dissolve.

Do-it-yourself head massage. Close your eyes and massage your head and neck in firm small circles. With your head and neck limp, massage the skull; then massage down along the neck vertebrae to the shoulder.

The 5-minute vacation. Put your feet up, close your eyes, breathe slowly and deeply, and let your muscles relax. Imagine yourself lying on a beach in the sun, or floating in the water, totally relaxed. Stay there for 5 minutes, for a refreshing, relaxing vacation you can take every day of the year!

Advanced Techniques of Relaxation

Abdominal breathing. Lie flat on your back; place one hand on your abdomen and one on your chest so you can feel yourself breathing with the abdomen, not the chest. Inhale deeply and slowly through the nostrils and expand the abdomen without pulling the air up to the chest. Keep your shoulders and chest relaxed and your back flat against the floor. Exhale slowly through the nostrils, pulling the abdomen to the back of the spine. Concentrate on your breath, feel the air going in and out.

Progressive relaxation. Lie on your back, close your eyes. Breathe in deeply through the nose; exhale as far as you can, releasing your breath very slowly. Starting with your feet, tense your muscles; then let go. Tense one foot, let it relax; tense the other foot, let it relax. Tense and relax each leg, your abdomen, chest, and shoulders; then all along your spine and back. Feel the muscles begin to loosen. Tighten your buttocks muscles and let them relax. Let your back go flat against the floor. Close and open your fists. Tense the muscles in each arm, let them relax. Shrug your shoulders, let them relax. Let your neck relax. Tense your facial muscles, let them relax. Let your jaw sag. Yawn. Let your scalp loosen. Let your eyes relax. Feel relaxation enveloping your entire body. As you breathe in and out, feel the tension leave you.

Meditation. The meditative state is similar to the first moments of falling asleep. Find a quiet place, sit in a comfortable position, and close your eyes. Take a deep, slow, long breath. Let calmness come into your body. Let your muscles relax and your mind drift.

There are many variations of meditation techniques. With some, you let your mind wander as it wishes; with others, you keep saying one word or phrase over and over, or you concentrate on your breathing. In "one-pointing" you contemplate a pleasant object, focusing your gaze on a lighted candle, a leaf, a flower, or still water. Some techniques combine movement with meditation.

You May Do Best to Get Professional Help

Many of these techniques, especially those of abdominal breathing and progressive relaxation, take professional help to attain full benefits. You may want to check with your family doctor, a psychologist, psychiatrist, local clinic, or university (or look in the Yellow Pages under "Stress Reduction") for instruction in these techniques for reducing tension. Some companies are now offering stress reduction workshops for their employees.

CHAPTER NINE

What Diet, Vitamins, and Minerals Can Do for Your Back

Our national diet has been so nutritionally poor that the government has linked it to at least six of the ten leading causes of death: heart disease, cancer, strokes, diabetes, hardening of the arteries, and cirrhosis of the liver. Poor diet can affect your back, too.

Bone is alive and always changing, consistently building up and breaking down its components. It vitally needs good nutrition. The right diet can provide the vitamins and minerals needed to make bones strong and keep them that way.

In addition, the right diet can help you lose weight if you're obese—one of the biggest causes of backache. You may be careful not to lift heavy things so that you don't strain your back, but if you are overweight, you lift a heavy weight every day. Having a potbelly puts a constant forward pull on struggling back muscles. It's a lever effect; for every pound of extra weight you have on your abdomen, it is estimated that you are putting as much as 5 pounds of pressure on your back. Ten pounds of extra weight up front can cause more strain on your lower back than can carrying around a bowling ball all day. The good news is that is can also work in reverse: for every pound you lose, you relieve 5 pounds of pressure from your back.

Excess weight not only strains your back directly, it also often keeps you from exercising. The more weight you have, the more you lie down, the more you lie down, the more you gain weight, the more you gain weight, the more problems you have with your back.

Obesity also alters body mechanics, and the constant struggle to maintain good posture makes back pain even worse. Obese patients more frequently have back trouble, more arthritis of the spine, and a longer period of recovery from back injuries. The faster you gain the weight, the more it seems to affect your back. In fact, most people who gain weight suddenly will develop back pain. If this is true in your case, pay special attention to the guidelines of our diet and exercise program so that you can get back to a better weight for you.

One patient, a 250-pound accountant from Georgia, had back surgery at the Institute that resulted in his being pain-free for six months. Then he put on an extra 30 pounds and his back started hurting all the time. X-rays showed that the surgery had worked, that there was no further disc damage. Once he was put on a diet, however, he lost those 30 pounds, and his pain went away.

Taking the time and effort to keep off excess weight before you have a back problem can significantly help to lower your risk of back pain, and if you already have back pain, it can be a tremendous advantage in helping you benefit from back treatments.

Whenever an overweight patient comes to the Institute, the first thing we tell that person is: "Get rid of excess weight!" This is one of the most important things you can do to get rid of back pain and to protect your back from future trouble.

The Back Pain/Overeating Cycle

People with back pain often react in one of two different ways in the way they eat. (1) They become depressed and because of the depression begin to ignore their nutrition, eating very little because of no appetite or eating unnutritious packaged food that needs little preparation. (Pain-killing drugs, too, can dull appetite and lead to bad eating habits.) Or (2) they become binge eaters. They gorge themselves, especially on carbohydrates, sugar, and chocolate, because they use food as a pacifier for their pain and depression. Since they often eat junk foods with little nutritional value, they not only gain weight, but can also be nutritionally undernourished.

It's a vicious cycle: the excess weight worsens the back pain, the pain and depression lead to less sensible eating habits and poor nutrition, poor nutrition means fewer body resources for combatting pain, the pain and depression worsen, and food intake becomes even more erratic.

The Better Back Diet

The following Better Back Diet will help you break the spiral.

This diet program is designed for three things: to help you be slim, to give you nutrients to help relieve pain and inflammation, and to help you overcome possible deficiencies in the vitamins and minerals that have been shown to be most related to preventing and overcoming back problems.

1. *Avoid sugar.* Read labels when you buy so you avoid any foods or drinks with hidden sugar. Watch for hidden sugars in such things as instant lemonade, canned fruits, and cereals.
2. *Avoid refined carbohydrates.* Don't eat such things as white bread, white rice, cakes, or cookies. Do eat whole grain foods instead.

3. *Avoid processed, imitation, and synthetic foods.* Do eat as wide a variety as you can of fresh fruits, salads, and vegetables. Buy them in season for maximum freshness.

4. *Limit fats and oils to moderate amounts.* (Don't eliminate them completely; you need adequate amounts for hormones, smooth skin, and natural lubrication.) Stop frying; rather, broil, steam, or stir-fry instead.

5. *Limit your intake of coffee, tea, and caffeine colas.* This is especially important if you tend to be tense, anxious, or irritable from caffeine, or if you have insomnia or urinary urgency. (Also be alert for medicines that contain caffeine.) Do drink plenty of water.

6. *Limit alcohol.* Excessive alcohol not only adds many calories, it is associated with higher risk of osteoporosis because it impairs calcium absorption and decreases the liver's ability to activate vitamin D.

7. *Limit your intake of red meats.* Do get some of your protein from fish, poultry, eggs, or cheese.

8. *Eat calcium-rich foods.* Milk, yogurt, and cheese are good sources of calcium, as are broccoli, dried peas and beans, and sardines with bones. Calcium-rich foods should not be eaten simultaneously with foods that inhibit calcium absorption, such as asparagus, beet greens, spinach, oatmeal, bran, and brown rice.

9. *Eat tryptophan-rich foods.* Tryptophan is an amino acid, one of the building blocks of protein that is present in most foods. Research has shown that increased levels of tryptophan in the diet increase serotonin levels in the brain, which can induce and prolong sleep, calm nerves, curb the appetite, and increase tolerance to pain—all of which are important to the person with an aching back. The following foods are good sources of tryptophan: veal, beef, lamb, chicken, turkey, fish, milk, eggs, cheese, and green vegetables.

10. *Eat foods high in vitamin C.* Vitamin C has a key role in the production of collagen, an important structural protein of the body, and experimental evidence indicates that it may play a role in bone mineralization. Researchers at the University of Texas Southwestern Medical Center just recently have shown that vitamin C also is effective at counteracting the LDL ("bad") form of cholesterol that can cause impaired circulation. Foods rich in vitamin C are citrus fruits, tomatoes, green peppers, parsley, dark green leafy vegetables, broccoli, cantaloupe, and strawberries.

Some Ways to Make the Diet Easy for Yourself

Start by eliminating two of your biggest offenders. Do you have a weakness for a particular fattening dessert? a sugary snack? a "comfort food" you turn to under stress? Decrease the amounts of two of these foods by limiting the number of times you have them during each month as well as the amount you eat of them each time. After you have the first two major offenders under control, find two other offenders and eat them only once or twice a month. Just getting a few high-fat, high-calorie foods under control if you are used to eating them often can make a significant change in your weight and your nutrition.

Don't keep candy, cookies, cakes, pies, and sugared drinks in the house.

Read labels and choose foods accordingly. (Ingredients are listed in order of the amounts in the food.)

Don't overcook food. In order to take advantage of their full nutritional value (and so that they'll be as tasty as possible, too!), eat vegetables garden-fresh and still crispy.

Cook with as little water as possible. Use leftover cooking water for soups or stews; use leftover vegetables in salads the next day instead of cooking them again and causing more nutrient loss.

Keep whatever vitamin and mineral supplements have been recommended to you on the kitchen counter at all times so that it's easy to grab them at the right times. (But don't take more than you should. Vitamins and minerals need to be in balance. One doctor, for example, found that some patients with chronic pain were suffering from vitamin A toxicity; their pain went away when they stopped taking vitamin A supplements.)

Set up nutritious snacks where everyone can easily reach them, both in the refrigerator and on the kitchen counter. Some good treats are: fruit juices, herbal tea, cottage cheese, yogurt, cheese, leftover fish and chicken, melon slices, carrot and celery sticks, cauliflower buds, radishes, cabbage chunks, green peppers, tomatoes, tangerines, apples, oranges, grape-fruits, bananas, dried apricots, dates, raisins, figs, prunes, whole wheat crackers, or whole grain bread. In the freezer you might have individual containers of frozen yogurt or popsicles of frozen juice.

Visit a health food store. See if there is anything there that appeals to you: papaya juice, sunflower seeds, nonsugared yogurt.

Change the proportions of your food groups. Have some kind of salad at every lunch and dinner, and make vegetables the largest portion on the plate and protein the smallest.

Go Ahead and Nibble

On this diet it's okay to nibble, even if you are trying to lose weight. Research with animals shows that animals fed many times a day gain less weight than do those fed the same total of food in only three meals. You may find you lose weight and feel better if you eat five little meals a day instead of three large ones.

However, if you nibble, make sure your snacks are not weight-producing sweets and starches. Instead of sugar for a lift, eat a salad or a protein snack of cheese, fowl, fish, beans, or nuts every few hours—it will give you long-lasting energy. This can help with irritability and tension too, which can be caused by wide fluctuations in sugar levels in the blood.

Why You May Need Certain Extra Vitamins and Minerals

Some physicians believe that our diets today are perfectly okay, that the food in the average diet has enough of the essential vitamins and minerals. Others—ourselves included—believe that current recommendations of vitamins and minerals given as the U.S. Recommended Daily Allowances (RDAs) are much lower than they should be. To assure optimum health and to eliminate many chronic, everyday symptoms, some higher amounts of vitamin and mineral supplements usually are necessary.

Whether a new diet and extra vitamins and minerals help *your* back depends on what the underlying cause of you backache is, how good or bad your present diet is, and whether your body for some reason (such as poor absorption) needs certain extra nutrients. Many patients, after using a no-sugar, no-refined-starches diet with increased amounts of vitamins and minerals, find that their backaches disappear within several weeks. For other patients, whose eating habits were good to start with, a new nutrition program makes no improvement. Each person has to make his or her own decision, preferably with the help of a doctor who is knowledgeable in nutrition.

With so many widely differing opinions on vitamin needs, it is difficult for a patient to know how to make the best decision. One way to get an objective answer is by an individualized laboratory test. Computer analysis of your diet can help to determine if you are getting enough vitamins. Hair mineral analysis and blood tests can help your doctor to analyze deficiencies or excesses of minerals in your body as well as whether the ratios of the minerals to each other are proper.

If these tests indicate that you have deficiencies, if you have other reasons for believing you have deficiencies, or if you have any chronic conditions in addition to your back trouble that are of concern to you, consult a doctor who has experience with nutrition medicine to learn whether you should be taking any more or less of certain nutrients.

In general, we recommend that anyone with a chronic back problem take a good vitamin supplement *that also includes minerals*, plus other extra supplements that their doctor might approve of, such as calcium or vitamin C.

The most recent research indicates a new concept: that bone health depends not just on calcium, but on many nutrients including vitamins B6, C, D and K; folic acid; and magnesium, manganese, boron, zinc, copper, strontium, and silicon. All these nutrients are essential to efficient formation and maintenance of bone and have been shown by a number of surveys to be frequently deficient in the typical diet today.

One of the excellent examples of the importance of these minerals is the case of a famous professional basketball player who had suffered many fractures that healed poorly. He was found to have osteoporosis *and* deficiencies in many minerals. In fact, no manganese whatsoever could be found in his blood. After six weeks of supplements, he could play basketball again.

Calcium Supplements

Calcium is essential for strong bones. Without it, your bones may soften and weaken, often fracturing from the slightest blow because they are so brittle. Indeed, a deficiency in calcium is one of the biggest factors in causing osteoporosis, the bone-weakening that often happens with aging.

Osteoporosis most commonly appears in women who are postmenopausal or who have undergone hysterectomies, but both men and women can get it. As the disease progresses, bones in the back, hips, and other areas lose calcium and phosphate salts and eventually become porous and brittle. In some cases the vertebrae of the spine get so brittle that the spine collapses on itself in a compression fracture, or a person can crack a rib just by turning in bed.

It can cause the fractures that occur so often in older people after minor falls, as well as "dowager's hump," and loss of height. In fact, often when a person falls down and breaks a hip, the hip actually broke *first* because it was so weak, *then* the person fell down (more about this on page 182). About one in four women and one in eight men have osteoporosis and the back pain that usually goes with it.

According to the U.S. Department of Agriculture, three out of every ten families have a calcium intake below the recommended minimum. You probably get enough calcium if you drink a lot of milk or eat a lot of cheese or lots of sardines with bones. A cup of yogurt has about 400 mg. Otherwise, researchers believe most adults should take calcium supplements throughout life. They are available in any drug or health food store. Calcium nitrate has been shown to be more effective than calcium carbonate. Buy supplements that also contain magnesium and zinc.

There are also some other bonus benefits from calcium/ magnesium supplements: your cholesterol levels will usually decrease, leg cramps often disappear, and there is often a lessening of irritability and fatigue. Statistical studies also show fewer cases of colon cancer in populations that have higher calcium intake, and 1991 studies from Framingham show a relationship also to heart disease: the lower the calcium, the higher the risk of heart attack.

Postmenopausal women should get 800–1,000 mg of calcium per day if they are taking estrogen, and 1,500 mg if they are not. (Loss of bone mass accelerates most rapidly at the hip and spine during the first four to eight years following menopause due to reduced production of the hormone estrogen, according to recent research by Dr. B. Lawrence Riggs of the Endocrine Research Unit of the Mayo Clinic.)

Current recommendations are that children need 800 mg of calcium daily (most children would get this much calcium if they drink milk regularly, but milk has too little magnesium), pregnant or nursing woman need 1,400–2,000 mg, and adult men need 1,000 mg daily.

For adolescence to midtwenties, 1,600 mg is recommended. This is because today's typical teenager's diet is low in calcium and high in phosphorus from consuming soft drinks and processed foods, possibly shortchanging the amount of bone they should be developing and setting them up for later osteoporosis.

Aging people, especially, need calcium supplements. They generally take in less calcium in the diet, and as people age, their calcium absorption capacity usually lessens.

In addition to calcium supplements, you may also need to have adequate vitamin D to increase absorption of calcium and facilitate new bone formation, so get plenty of sunshine. (Any vitamin D supplements should be regulated by a physician since excessive amounts can be toxic and actually cause *decreased* bone mass.) There is some evidence that excess salt in the diet or large amounts of protein can increase calcium loss, so don't let them dominate your diet.

You should not have a daily intake of more than 5,000 units of vitamin A, since more than that can stimulate bone loss.

Exercise is also vital to strengthen bones and help prevent osteoporosis. Stress decreases calcium absorption and increases calcium excretion.

There also can be medical factors involved in calcium needs. Diuretics (often used for high blood pressure), antacids, anticonvulsants, and other medicines, for example, can increase the need for calcium and other minerals. Prolonged use of cortisone or its derivatives can lead to severe calcium loss, to the point that patients can run a high risk of bone fracture.

Most doctors recommend that anyone taking cortisone should also take calcium supplements, along with vitamin D, to prevent the bone degeneration.

Bone that is immobilized also loses calcium. A person who has had an arm or leg in a cast for several weeks will have as much as a 50 percent loss of calcium. When the bone is no longer immobilized and is exercised and used for weight-bearing, it recovers. (This is why people with osteoporosis are no longer put into braces. It isn't protection they need, but exercise and calcium to speed the healing of bone and to prevent fractures.)

How can you tell if you have a calcium deficiency? Your *dentist* may be the first to know! Often the jawbone shows the first signs of demineralization. If your dentist finds signs of bone thinning, you may be able to take steps to correct the calcium and other deficiencies before your spinal vertebrae show the same signs of thinning. (Calcium supplements will usually also decrease gum inflammation.)

Bones in the fingers also may show early signs of mineral loss when their density is measured by X ray. However, the earliest indicator is found in hair mineral analysis since hair reflects changes in calcium content even before bone or teeth do.

Note: Some doctors claim that excessive calcium can cause kidney stones, and others say that taking estrogen and calcium can increase the risk of developing gallstones, so if you have a history of kidney stones or gallstones, consult with your physician before taking these supplements. Giving extra magnesium with the calcium will usually solve the problem.

Tryptophan Foods

Does tryptophan really help counteract pain? Apparently so. Dr. Robert Pollack, author of *The Pain-Free Tryptophan Diet* (Warner 1986), and Dr. Samuel Seltzer, Temple University pain researcher, used carefully controlled diets and tryptophan supplementation and found that it was indeed often possible to diminish long-lasting pain with tryptophan.

Dr. Richard Wurtman of the Massachusetts Institute of Technology and his wife, Dr. Judith Wurtman, also showed that carbohydrate is a key factor in helping to get tryptophan to the brain. When you eat carbohydrates, insulin is released into the blood stream, and the insulin is the aid to tryptophan getting into the brain.

Just eating tryptophan-rich foods doesn't necessarily ensure that tryptophan reaches the brain, because there is much competition from other amino acids at the blood-brain barrier. Eating carbohydrates at the same time as tryptophan foods helps to get the tryptophan across the blood-brain barrier and into the brain, where it can do some good.

There are two other ways to increase the utilization of tryptophan. One is to limit fat in the diet. The other is to eat foods high in vitamin B$_3$ (niacin) and vitamin B$_6$ (pyridoxine).

There are other benefits to a high-tryptophan diet. One of the reasons that exercise is beneficial—in addition to strengthening muscles and getting rid of fat—is that exercise has the ability to reduce pain by promoting the release by the brain of a chemical called *endorphin*. Endorphin is a natural pain-reliever, and as it surges into the bloodstream, it increases the tolerance to all kinds of pain—including back pain. Tryptophan also increases the amount of endorphins in your body and gives significant mood elevation. Patients suffering from depression say it often disappears when eating high amounts of tryptophan. You also may feel more rested since tryptophan can improve sleep.

In 1989, there were some side effects found to be connected to some tryptophan supplements, and at the time of the writing of this book, tryptophan supplements had been taken off the market. Since then, however, the FDA has announced that the side effects were due to contamination from one manufacturer. When the supplements are again available to purchase, you can discuss with your doctor whether you should take them. Meanwhile, you can get your tryptophan naturally from the foods we have listed.

Vitamin C

The mechanism is not clear, but recent research indicates that vitamin C seems to counteract back pain. Several studies indicate that large doses of vitamin C relieved pain and increased mobility significantly in many patients. For example, Dr. J. Greenwood, Jr., reported in the *Medical Annals of the District of Columbia* that he gave vitamin C to more than 500 patients who had low back pain due to sprain, disc injury, disc surgery, or degenerative disc disease. In a great number of patients, back pain was helped by the vitamin C, recurred when treatment was stopped, and improved again with resumption of vitamin C treatment. A significant number of patients with early disc problems were able to avoid surgery after taking vitamin C, and those who required surgery appeared to have a smoother convalescence, Dr. Greenwood said.

If a diet is deficient enough in vitamin C, scurvy can occur. The capillaries become fragile, causing hemorrhages into the joints, muscle, and skin; bones become weak; dentine and enamel fail to form; the jawbone begins to be resorbed; and gum tissue becomes inflamed and spongy.

Special Advice for Premenstrual Backache

Backache frequently goes along with tension, fatigue, and irritability during the premenstrual periods. To help alleviate the problem, some doctors recommend that in the days before a woman's menstrual period, she eliminate salt, sugar, and carbohydrates from the diet to produce water loss.

Nutrition aids that sometimes help to reduce premenstrual problems are: vitamin A, vitamin B complex, vitamin C, calcium, vitamin E, lecithin, wheat germ, and protein snacks every few hours.

Hormones sometimes help, and many women on birth-control pills say they no longer have backache or other premenstrual problems.

Advice on Special Helps After Menopause

Backache can sometimes appear after menopause, along with a loss of muscle tone and sometimes is misdiagnosed as arthritis. The calcium level also usually drops greatly when ovarian hormones decrease.

Some nutritionists claim that hot flashes, night sweats, leg cramps, irritability, and backache can sometimes disappear in a few days by taking calcium supplements plus a small amount of vitamin D or fish oil to assimilate the calcium.

The B vitamins can also help to overcome jangled nerves and resulting tensed muscles in the neck and back. Eat lots of liver, wheat germ, or brewer's yeast, or take properly balanced vitamin B-complex tablets. Lecithin, which is a vitamin B derivative, may help too, because it aids the body to use calcium and maintain a hormone balance.

Estrogen is recommended by many physicians to help prevent osteoporosis with its usual accompanying backache. Estrogen-treated menopausal woman have a much lower incidence of wrist and hip fractures, and of vertebral fractures.

Taking estrogen pills has been shown to counteract weakening of bones and help low back pain, as well as bring relief from hot flashes and dry vaginal membranes. Women should see a doctor about starting estrogen therapy and ask that the dose prescribed be as low as possible.

Many women find that if they take 1 to 5 mg of folic acid,

symptoms of backaches and vaginal dryness disappear even without estrogen. Folic acid has also been reported to increase sexual desire and to improve joint mobility and eliminate some arthritis pain. In the United States a prescription is needed for these amounts, but not in Canada.

The Nightshade Foods—"Good" and "Bad"

Many patients believe that they experience pain after ingesting foods in the nightshade group, especially if these people have an arthritis-type pain. The nightshade group includes tomatoes, white potatoes, green peppers, paprika, and eggplant. The Arthritis Foundation, however, says there is no scientific evidence for this.

Fish oils appear to be good for helping to prevent flare-ups of rheumatoid arthritis. Dr. Jack Kremer of Albany Medical College, New York, reported in *Arthritis and Rheumatism* (June 1990) that patients with this type of arthritis had improvement with less stiffness and pain after six months of taking fish oil capsules. The benefits of omega-3 fish oil in rheumatoid arthritis have also been shown by researchers at Harvard and in Australia.

We have no experience with either of these but see no harm in eliminating nightshade foods from your diet for several weeks to see if there is any effect on your back pain, and then after waiting several weeks, adding fish oil capsules or fish-containing omega-3s—such as salmon, tuna, halibut, and sardines—to your diet.

CHAPTER TEN

When You Go to the Doctor

Most people with bad backs do not go to the doctor soon enough. They may get so used to periodic back pain that they accept it as being normal, or they may think that nothing can be done.

The truth is, if a slightly bad back is not attended to, the chances are strong that the condition will get worse. And some back pain can be a sign of serious disease that could be life threatening if not attended to properly; an aortic aneurysm, for example, can cause back pain. Perhaps your back has been hurting off and on for quite a while now, and recently it seems to be worse. When should you get professional help? Whenever back pain is severe, or even when mild discomfort is constant or frequently reappears, a doctor should be seen for diagnosis and advice.

When to Go to the Doctor

If you have been putting off going to the doctor, read the following list. If any of these circumstances applies to you, stop procrastinating and see your doctor.

- Your backache persists and is getting no better.
- Your backaches are occurring more frequently or severely.
- You have pain that radiates down an arm or leg, even if you don't have back pain.
- You have numbness or tingling or a feeling of weakness in your arms or legs.
- You have difficulty with bladder or bowel function.
- Pain wakes you up in the middle of the night.
- Your backache does not improve a little with a day of rest.
- There is a severe limitation of movement.
- Your neck is so stiff that your head cannot be lowered toward the chest.
- You have other symptoms with the backache, such as loss of appetite, weight loss, or fever.

The most ominous sign—that a backache could be due to aortic aneurysm, for example—is if a back pain seems to come on suddenly out of nowhere without any obvious cause; or if you have unrelenting or progressively worse pain that is not helped by rest; or if the pain is excruciatingly bad in bed at night. If you have any of these symptoms, you should see your doctor immediately for X rays and laboratory tests.

Who Are You Going to See?

Since there's no single cause to back pain and no single cure, there is no one specialist who is right for every case. The following are typical of the people you can go to for help. If it is appropriate, one doctor can refer you to another for different specialized treatment. One good approach is to go to a back center, sometimes located in a hospital or clinic and sometimes operating independently, where you will find surgeons, internists, psychiatrists, physical therapists, and others working together as a team.

If you don't feel confident in one practitioner's treatment, go to a second doctor and compare his or her recommendations. It is usually best not to say you are coming for a "second opinion," but to come as a fresh patient; however, tell the new physician of any previous treatments and their outcomes.

Family practitioner. A good place to start if you have a back problem, since your family doctor knows your medical history. Your family practitioner can refer you to a specialist if appropriate.

Orthopedic surgeon (orthopedist). A physician who, after medical school, an internship, and training in general surgery, spends three to four years in a residency in the specialty of treating bone and muscle problems. Although an orthopedic surgeon is basically a surgeon, he or she also used various nonsurgical treatments for the bones and joints.

Neurologist. A physician who specializes in the treatment of disorders affecting the nervous system, including the spine and spinal nerves. A neurologist uses nonsurgical methods.

Physiatrist. A physician who specializes in physical medicine. A physiatrist does not perform surgery and usually employs a physical therapist to give exercises, heat treatment, ultrasound therapy, and so on. A physiatrist frequently is also involved in rehabilitation medicine to improve and restore function.

Osteopathic physician. A physician who has gone to a school of osteopathy, which awards the doctor of osteopathy (D.O.) degree rather than the M.D. degree. A D.O. may be a general practitioner or a specialist. Osteopathic training emphasizes the musculoskeletal, circulatory, and nervous systems and uses manipulation as a means of diagnosis and treatment in addition to the use of drugs, surgery, and other therapy.

Chiropractor. One who has training in chiropractor school but does not have a degree in medicine and cannot prescribe medicines or perform surgery. Chiropractors believe that misalignments of the vertebrae of the spine can produce a variety of symptoms that may often then be helped by manipulative techniques to put them back into proper alignment. Chiropractors who belong to the International Chiropractors Association (ICA) usually use X rays to locate misalignments and then use manipulations to correct them. Those in the American Chiropractic Association (ACA) usually also use heat, hydrotherapy, ultrasound, acupuncture, and other techniques to aid in diagnosis and treatment.

How to Work With Your Doctor

First, to find a doctor to treat your back, don't just walk into an emergency room or search the Yellow Pages. Talk to other patients who have had a similar problem and see who they recommend or, if you have a family physician, get a recommendation from him or her.

Then visit the doctor to see if he or she fills your needs and if you have good communications. Is the doctor willing to answer your questions? Are you simply told that you will have to learn to live with your pain, or does the doctor outline a program of diagnosis and possible treatment for your problem that you can work on together?

Talk to your doctor. Don't be intimidated by big words and medical terminology. Ask the doctor to explain things in detail. Never pretend to understand when you don't—you're apt to lose in the long run.

When you go for the first visit, be organized in discussing your problem. The more specific you can be in telling your doctor about your symptoms, the faster he or she can make a diagnosis and get started with proper treatment.

Take along your Self-testing Questionnaire (page 128). Be sure you tell the doctor of current medications, allergies, past surgeries, and any family history of back problems.

Write down the advice and instructions your doctor tells you, *in the office, while he is telling you.* Even the most intelligent, best organized person, within minutes of walking out of the office, seems to go blank on remembering all of the doctor's instructions.

When the doctor recommends a treatment, make sure that the treatment is explained, along with any potential risks or side effects, and ask about alternatives that might be available.

Facts to Know Before You Go

The more information you can bring to your doctor about your back problem, the more easily he or she can find the cause of your problem and the right treatment. For example, if the pain is low back pain with no pain in your arms or legs and you lifted something heavy or did some heavy yard work or had been in a car accident, it's likely you have a strained muscle—the most common cause of back injuries—and the pain will usually be gone in a few days with physical therapy and rest. If you are a woman with osteoporosis and the pain is strong and occurred suddenly, it's likely to be a collapsed vertebrae—the second most common cause of back pain. If there is pain radiating to the arm or leg, it is likely to be a bulging or ruptured disc.

What follows is a list of questions for you to think about before you go to the doctor, so that you can have the answers ready. You can even copy the questions directly from the book, write the answers, and give the written answers to your doctor to study and put with your other records. Pay attention to how your pain affects your daily functioning, and how it affects your family life, job, leisure activities, sleep patterns, sexual functioning, and ability to walk, bend, sit. Also pay attention to what makes your pain better or worse.

Discuss all your symptoms, even minor ones. This is no time to give in to false modesty or pretend that you are a superperson with no problems. Tell your doctor everything, even if it is embarrassing. No matter how embarrassing it may be to you, he or she probably has heard it before. Every clue could be important.

Don't wait for your doctor to ask you about something—volunteer information. And if you have a hunch as to what the cause of your back problem might be, or a fear about something, discuss it.

One more important thing: When your doctor gives you advice, follow it. Studies show that as many as 60 percent of the people who go to physicians ignore their advice. If some treatment, especially a medicine, does not seem to be working or is causing a side effect, call your doctor so he or she can change the medicine, the dosage, or time you take the medicine. Do not stop on your own without discussing it with your doctor.

Self-testing Questionnaire

1. What is your chief complaint about your back?
2. What other related or even seemingly unrelated symptoms do you have?
3. When did you first notice the pain, stiffness, or other symptoms?
4. Did it start suddenly, or did you gradually become aware of it?
5. How do you think the problem was produced?
6. Had you been ill in any other way when it started?
7. Had you been doing anything unusual before it began that may have led to strain or injury?
8. When does it bother you most (in the morning, during the day, at the end of the day, at night, with coughing, sneezing, straining, fatigue, certain movements)?
9. Is the pain sharp, aching, dull, throbbing, deep, burning, cramping, stabbing, shooting? Is there tingling or numbness?
10. Is it steady or does it come and go? How long does it last?
11. Is it in one spot or does it seem to spread down the arm or leg or into the hip?
12. Does the pain seem to be related to certain activities, such as having sexual intercourse, watching television, driving the car, engaging in a sport, doing certain work? Is it worse when you stand? sit? bend? lift? drive?
13. Has the discomfort affected your sleep? breathing? appetite? elimination? work? hobbies? relationships?
14. Are there things you can't do because of your back?
15. What medications do you take?
16. Have you ever had a similar problem? or any other neck, back, hip, leg, or foot problems?
17. What treatments did you have for any of these previous problems?
18. What treatments have you had, if any, for your present problem?
19. What have you found that helps relieve the problem?
20. What kind of work do you do? Does it involve standing or sitting for long periods or heavy lifting?
21. Do you consider yourself a tense person? Do you tend to frequently get angry or be depressed?

22. Is there anything else you would like your doctor to know about your problem?

Physical Examination Techniques
That Your Doctor May Use

The function of the examination is to determine where your pain is coming from—what is generating the pain. It could be originating from the joints, bones, muscles, discs, or nerves.

The doctor will check your body for balance and symmetry, noting your posture and how you walk or sit, such as listing to one side. You may be asked to bend forward, backward, and sideways or to bend and twist in various directions—much like the self-tests at the beginning of this book—so that the doctor can check to see if there is any limitation in your motion, or pain with certain movements. You may be checked along your spine for areas of heat, redness, sweating, patches of hair, swellings, nodules, tenderness.

Muscles may be checked for weakness or spasm, and whether they are equal on both sides. Your reflexes will be checked to determine if there is nerve damage, and your skin will be checked for sensory loss. You may be checked to see if you can feel vibrations from a tuning fork or pricks from a pin.

The doctor may "palpate" your back, feeling your muscles; checking for twitch response, painful knots, or trigger points; and checking the intervals between vertebrae and how easily you bend in different directions.

The doctor will also probably do the Straight-Leg Raising Test, in which you lie or sit on the examining table, and the doctor raises one leg with the other leg straight, and then flexes your foot or big toe. If there is pain that goes up the hip or back with these maneuvers, it indicates that certain spinal nerves are involved in your back pain.

The examiner may also do the Flip Test, in which you sit on the edge of the table, the knee is extended, and if you have tight hamstrings or tight back muscles, you will involuntarily lean back. The doctor may also have you push against resistance when he holds down your foot or leg. There is also the Bent Knee Test, the Neck Flexion Test, and other tests that help to pinpoint which areas of your spine are involved in causing you pain.

If your back pain radiates down into your arms or legs or hips or you have a burning or other strange sensation, it is likely that you have a spur or a bulging spinal disc pushing against a spinal nerve going to that area. According to where you feel pain, the doctor can determine what spinal nerve is involved and thus tell at what level the problem is located on your spine. We will tell you how to figure out these nerve pathways yourself in the section on disc problems (pages 185–189). It can be one of the most important keys of all to knowing the cause of your back pain.

The doctor will also measure the circumference of each thigh and each calf. This is to find if there has been any atrophy of the muscles, which could indicate a disc problem or other muscle or nerve disorder. Differences of ¼ inch or more in the calves and ½ inch or more in the thighs are considered significant. Smaller differences are disregarded. He or she will also probably check to see if one leg is cooler to the touch than the other, which often indicates nerve or blood vessel involvement.

All these methods help the physician to determine the specific problem areas.

Simple Causes You Might Not Think of

Part of the diagnostic workup will include checking for small, seemingly minor, things, but often they are the cause of backache. Perhaps you sit in a draft at work, or you have a saggy mattress, a chair that isn't right, or shoes that need replacing. The wrong bra can cause upper back pain in a woman with heavy breasts.

Short-Leg Syndrome

One leg being shorter than the other is a common—and often overlooked—cause of backache. Often the difference is so slight you are not even aware of it. Only a ¼-inch difference between the right and left legs can tilt the pelvis just enough to affect the spine and work the muscles harder on one side of the back, causing strain and backache that can become worse and worse with the years. It can be corrected easily in most cases with a simple heel lift. This was part of President John Kennedy's back problem, and he wore a lift in one shoe.

Short-Seatedness

Some persons spend more time sitting than standing, and their problem may be an uneven pelvis. The answer to this is to put lifts under one buttock when you sit. A pad is used on the smaller side of the pelvis. Some patients permanently attach a pad to one side of their car seat or chair at work.

Any lift should be carefully supervised because of the body's ability to adapt or compensate. Done incorrectly, it might create a problem in some other part of the spine and body.

Fat Wallets and Keys

If you have pain in the hip, upper leg, or buttocks, your wallet may be too thick.

One patient who traveled constantly by auto had been troubled for 14 months by "sciatica" before his doctor noticed the wallet he carried on the painful side. It was 1½ inches thick, packed with credit cards. Transferring the wallet to an inner coat pocket gave complete relief.

It Could Be Your Feet

If your back hurts, consider seeing a podiatrist (also called chiropodist) as part of the team to give you a strong back. Fallen arches (flat feet) can cause pain in the legs and back. (You probably have fallen arches if your feet seem to be completely flat on the bottom and no arch is visible on the side. You can test for flat feet by walking with wet feet on newspapers and looking at your footprints to see if there is a curve on the inner side of your footprint or not. You can also use your footprints to see if your muscles are balanced and you walk correctly, or whether your gait is abnormal.

A NORMAL FOOT   FALLEN ARCH

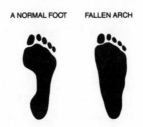

If there is a problem with your feet or legs, the podiatrist may prescribe exercises to strengthen the muscles of the feet, or may use corrective padding or arch supports to get your feet properly balanced so that you can walk with an even gait and avoid the imbalances that cause foot—and back—strain. (Don't do this on your own; you could make your condition worse and increase back pain by putting certain muscles under stress. Even when a professional puts in wedges or pads, watch carefully for a few weeks to see if your feet and back are improved, or if you develop any new aches and pains.)

If you have fallen arches and are overweight, you should lose weight to take the strain off your feet. Sometimes it is beneficial to use shock-absorbing insoles in the shoes to help prevent "heel-strike shock," when your heel hits the ground as you walk and sends shock waves to the legs and back. Some-times a heel cup will do it.

Bunions, ingrown toenails, and other painful problems of your feet can also cause back pain because you walk abnormally and force muscles out of balance.

Fitness Machines for Testing

Your doctor may want to test you on several fitness machines, some of which you may already be familiar with, such as treadmill, bicycle, and stair-climbing tests. Or the strength of your back muscles may be tested on special testing systems made by Biodex, Kin-Com, Cybex, or Loredan. You perform certain maneuvers with extensor and flexor muscles for a number of repetitions, and your performance is compared to normal levels.

A new apparatus is the Medex computerized equipment, developed by Arthur Jones, who also invented Nautilus exercise equipment. With the Medex machine, you sit in a large chair, where pads keep your pelvic area in place while you push against resistance. A computer records the strength and stamina of the work that can be done by the lumbar muscles in your back.

The Medex system is able to test for back weakness and injury. It is also useful for strengthening back muscles.

David Lehrman, M.D., director of the Lehrman Back Center in Miami, Florida, is developing a fleet of back-test vans to bring the Medex machines to industrial companies to identi-fy employees who are susceptible to back injury *before* injury occurs.

Two Tests You May Not Have Heard of

The Valsalva Test
This test increases the pressure within the body. To perform

the test, you bear down as if you were moving your bowels and at the same time hold your breath. The test is positive if you feel an increase in pain in the neck, upper back, or shoulder. It may indicate a herniated disc or tumor in the spinal canal.

Spine Distraction Test

This test is to determine if symptoms might be caused by arthritis of the spine or the vertebrae pushing down on some nerve roots and to see if stretching the spine by traction might be of some benefit in relieving the pain.

To perform the spine distraction test, the doctor places the open palm of one hand under the chin and the other hand under the back of the head and gradually and gently lifts the head, widening the spaces between the vertebral joints of the spine and relieving pressure.

Nerve and Muscle Studies

Tests may be done to evaluate nerves and muscles by electrically stimulating nerves and then recording the resulting nerve and muscle electrical activity. How fast the nerve impulses go helps to determine if there is nerve or muscle damage.

Electromyography (EMG) is sometimes done. For this test, a very thin needle is inserted into a muscle. Measurements are made of the electrical activity of the muscle at rest and as the patient contracts the muscle. This test can show changes in the electrical charges of muscle cells following injury.

Visualization Tests

There are many techniques to give your physician a better idea of what is happening inside your body structurally. Some are better for visualizing the bones, others for viewing muscles and ligaments and other soft tissue. Some of the techniques, such as the myelogram, are invasive, that is, they involve penetrating your body with an injection or other procedure, and others are noninvasive, such as X-ray or magnetic resonance imaging.

There is one thing that you must realize about all these techniques: they may show a spur, or an old compression fracture that has healed or other anatomical sign, *but this may not be the actual cause of your back pain.* An estimated one-third of the time, people have these kinds of "problems," but they have no pain because of them. You and your physician have to decide together what findings are significant in your particular case.

Here are the major visualization techniques currently used by back specialists.

X Rays

X-ray study will not tell the doctor as much as he or she might wish when it comes to back pain, but it can still be helpful by revealing a bone abnormality of the spine or osteoarthritic changes. A ruptured disc cannot be seen on an X ray, but sometimes the X ray can show narrowing of the spaces between the discs of the spine that may be an indication of trouble. If your doctor takes X rays, they will be made from several different angles in an attempt to visualize as much as possible of what is going on. X-ray studies are particularly helpful in finding small compression fractures of parts of the vertebrae. If these are suspected, follow-up X rays are usually taken six to eight weeks later to confirm the diagnosis and progress of healing.

X rays will not expose problems with muscles and other soft tissue, but they can help to rule out possible causes of your back pain, such as arthritis, kidney or lung disease, or bone damage.

Children and pregnant women should avoid X rays unless there are very urgent reasons for having them taken.

Magnetic Resonance Imaging

Magnetic resonance imaging (MRI) was introduced as a new technique to physicians just a few years ago, and it has already become a major tool in the diagnosis of muscle and bone disorders. Its chief advantage over other imaging techniques is that it shows soft tissues very well. It also does not require radiation or injections, as do some other techniques.

MRI uses a strong magnetic field, radio waves, and a computer to get highly detailed images of soft tissues and show the condition of your muscles, ligaments, tendons, cartilage, blood vessels, and other soft tissues, even bone marrow. It can also show areas of swelling, hemorrhage, or hidden bone fractures. X rays can't see through bone; MRI *can* see through bone to show pictures of soft tissue in any plane of any body part. The images are amazingly clear, almost as though the doctor were looking directly at the tissue.

You lie on a table and are slid into a tunnel-like machine. The procedure takes from 30 to 60 minutes. Some people are bothered by being confined in the apparatus and find it helpful to take a tranquilizer before the procedure. An attendant is with you at all times and is able to talk to you.

You shouldn't have magnetic resonance imaging if you are pregnant or if you have a cardiac pacemaker, metal fragments in your eyes from an accident, or metallic surgical implants (be sure to tell your doctor and the technician).

Computerized Tomography Scanning (CT or CAT Scan)

A CAT scan uses X rays that take cross sections of the body, so that structures deep within the tissue can be visualized. The X rays are usually taken in a series 1 to 3 minutes apart. Results are laid out by computer for the physician to see and interpret.

These cross-section views of the spine and spinal canal can show narrowing of the spinal canal and abnormalities and injuries of the vertebrae that cannot be seen on a regular X ray or a myelogram.

Sometimes a CAT scan is done with a fluid injected intravenously to increase the contrast.

Myelography

Because of its dangerous side effects and the need for a stay in the hospital, myelography is now only used when there is a special need such as locating a tumor. It can show a tumor of the spinal cord that might be mimicking symptoms of disc disease. For almost all other testing, it has been replaced by magnetic resonance.

In myelography a lumbar puncture is performed, inserting a needle between the vertebrae into the spinal canal. A small amount of cerebrospinal fluid is removed, a contrast medium is injected, and fluoroscope and X-ray pictures are taken of the spinal cord area.

After the test, the head must always be kept higher than the rest of the body so the contrast medium does not run into the head. There may be headaches, nausea, dizziness, or other reactions during or after the test (which should be reported promptly to the physician).

Bone Scanning

Radioisotope studies are sometimes done to study bone tissue. A radioactive chemical is injected into a vein and monitored by a scanner. The scan detects increased metabolic activity that could mean a healing fracture, some kinds of infections, and other problems. How and where the bone becomes radioactive also makes it possible for the doctor to spot a possible cancer or to determine if an injury to the bone is new or old.

Thermography

This technique, sometimes called infrared thermography or

neurothermography, doesn't really visualize body organs, but uses a very sensitive electronic infrared scanning camera to pick up differences in body activity by small differences in skin temperature. Temperatures of the skin should be symmetrical on a person's two sides. When there is a difference between the two sides, it usually indicates a trouble spot.

Sometimes thermography will reveal a place where there is reduced blood flow or injury to certain nerves when previous tests made it appear that the patient's pain had no organic source.

Laboratory Studies

Your doctor will probably take blood and urine samples. Tests for sedimentation rate of the blood and blood cell counts will show if there is an inflammatory process at work in the body. A high uric acid level in the blood indicates gout; other blood tests may indicate the possible presence of arthritis or cancer.

Psychological Tests

Since there often is a psychological factor involved in back pain, even when there is a physical cause, your doctor may want to do some psychological tests. Some patients have a lowered pain tolerance because of a depressed condition that they don't even realize that they have. Others may have hidden tension that is resulting in constriction of blood flow to back muscles or in muscle tightness.

However, it is important to realize that just because there were no physical causes found for a person's back pain, it does not necessarily mean that there is a psychological cause. It may just be that the physical cause has not yet been found. But you should consider the *possibility* that psychological factors are involved.

If your doctor thinks that tension may be playing a role in your back problem, he or she may have you tested with a biofeedback machine. It will monitor your pulse rate, sweat-gland activity, temperature, muscle tension, and other body reactions that reflect how tense your body is and how well you are able to relax.

Tests used to study personality traits are *not* usually considered accurate for predicting a psychological cause of back pain, and we use them only occasionally. A test more often used in back clinics is the Mensana Clinic Back Pain Test, developed by Dr. Nelson Hendler of Stevenson, Maryland, to measure the impact of pain on the patient's life and to help predict which patients have actual physical causes to their back pain and which do not.

How to Find Out What Your Doctor Really Means

It is important that you know about your condition in detail and understand exactly what to do. Remember, talk to your doctor, ask questions, take notes, make sure you understand instructions completely.

The following definitions will give the basic parts of the common medical words you might encounter when you talk to your doctor. By breaking a word down to its component parts you can usually figure out the meaning of most medical words.

When your doctor says . . .	*This is what he really means . . .*
arthro-	joint
-itis	inflammation
Arthritis	inflammation of a joint
costa-	rib

When your doctor says...	This is what he really means...
Intercostal	between the ribs
coxa-	hip
-algia	pain
Coxalgia	pain in the hips
myo-	muscle
Myositis	inflammation of muscles
osteo-	bone
-otomy	to cut open
Osteotomy	cutting into a bone
plasty-	repair
Arthroplasty	repair of a joint

How to Read the Prescription Your Doctor Gives You

Rx	means	prescription
Sig	means	label
ac	means	before meals
ad lib	means	whenever you want
bid	means	twice a day
cc	means	cubic centimeter
dr	means	dram
extr	means	extract
gm	means	gram
gr	means	grain
mg	means	milligram
qd	means	every day
qid	means	four times a day
tid	means	three times a day

CHAPTER ELEVEN

Up-to-Date Treatments Your Doctor May Prescribe

Scott, a famous designer of men's accessories, went to the doctor after he fell 10 feet from a ladder and hurt his back. Bob, an early-retired millionaire, went to the doctor when he pulled a back muscle jerking up a stubborn garage door. Computer programmer Brenda went because of off-and-on back pain that just wouldn't go away no matter what she did.

The cases are typical of the different causes of back pain. Most cases of backache fall into one of three broad categories: muscle strain, disc disease, or damage from long-term wear and tear on the spinal structure. Treatments will vary depending on whether pain is short term or long-lasting, and on what caused it. But no matter what the cause, with today's new research, you should no longer have to hear a doctor say "You'll just have to live with it."

If you have a sagging mattress, poor posture, heavy lifting at work, a fat wallet in your pocket, one leg shorter than the other, or other straightforward situation that could be causing your backache, then your treatment may be as simple as correcting the trouble-causing situation. However, often more than that is needed.

Sometimes the Institute sees a back pain patient who works two jobs or works much overtime; eats mostly cookies, candies, cakes, pies, TV dinners, and other junk foods; drinks coffee all day, chain smokes cigarettes; doesn't exercise; slouches in front of the TV all evening—and wonders what's wrong with his or her body that could cause a backache.

Most back pains involve more than a simple cause and a simple cure. That's why you need a total program—and why you may need to try different treatments to see what works best for you.

Even for the same cause of backache, one treatment may work in one person and not in another. As you go through any back treatment program, you need to be very observant as to the treatments that work best in your particular case.

But remember as you try different treatments: about one out of three back pain episodes will spontaneously be resolved in a week whether treated or not. It is also important to remember that, if not treated, episodes of back pain usually occur over and over again. So the important thing is not just treating the episode of pain, but preventing recurrence of the pain and stopping the progression of the problem.

In Chapter 3, we discussed the techniques to use at home to give immediate help to an aching back—muscle-relieving positions, heat applications, hot tub soaks, ice applications. In this chapter, we tell you about some of the additional things a professional health expert might do or recommend to help your back.

But remember the most important aid of all: your exercise program. You need to keep up your exercise program, and if necessary, help solve your problem by losing weight, improving your posture, becoming a nonsmoker to improve your circulation, and learning to manage stress better—even with the treatments described in this chapter that your doctor may use.

Bedrest

Bedrest is usually the single most important thing for a painful episode of an acute back strain. It reduces stress and prevents further strain. It also relieves pressure on spinal nerves because, when weight is taken off the spine, the discs between the vertebrae tend to expand and increase the space between the vertebrae. (Astronauts on return from space are taller because their spines have expanded with no gravity.) Sitting in a chair does not give the same kind of relief.

The value of bedrest was proven by Drs. S. W. Weisel and R. H. Rothman in a study reported in the journal *Clinical Orthopedics* in 1979 on acute low back pain in 80 servicemen. Half were kept at complete bedrest, and half were kept ambulatory. The bedrest group were able to return to full duty 50 percent faster and experienced less pain than did the ambulatory group.

In our experience at the GCOC Institute, two days of bedrest for back pain is the maximum that should be taken. Any longer and many people's muscles begin to weaken. Although there is some controversy among doctors as to how much bedrest is best for back treatment, most agree that for every week of bedrest, two weeks of special therapy is needed to strengthen atrophied muscles.

If you rest in bed, you should stay in bed except when you need to go to the bathroom. To ease your back the most, lie flat on your back with a pillow under your knees or lie on your side with a pillow between your knees. Try the Flat Pelvic Tilt position (Exercise 3 in Chapter 4) or any variation of it that makes you more comfortable.

However, remember that in most cases rest should be used as treatment only for right-now *acute* conditions, not long-term *chronic* ones. The back with a chronic condition needs exercise to stretch and strengthen it.

If You Have Muscle Spasm

When you have a sprain or strain, or any injury of your back, you probably also have muscle spasm, with the muscles tightening in constant contraction. The symptoms of a spasm include pain, stiffness, and reduced mobility. Usually, if you touch the area, the affected muscle seems taut and hard, or there may be swelling, and applying pressure usually makes the pain worse.

However, even though a muscle spasm is painful, it serves a purpose—the body is using the spasm as a splint to protect the injured area and prevent further aggravations of the injury.

The first aim of treatment for spasm of a back muscle is bedrest in a flat position to allow the muscles to relax and return from their spasm to their normal resting length.

If you are going to stay in bed, you can use a muscle relaxant, but otherwise do not. The tightness may go away, but injury may be done. Muscle relaxants usually cause drowsiness (you definitely shouldn't drive if you've taken any).

The GCOC philosophy is to avoid medications as much as possible. There are other ways to help relax muscles to help break the cycle of muscle spasm and help alleviate pain. For treatment of an acute strain or after surgery, we recommend applying ice. For chronic problems that have been present for a longer time, wet heat is usually best.

Some physicians use tranquilizers as a muscle relaxant. The physicians at GCOC do not. We find that tranquilizers are of very little help in managing back pain and are contraindicated for backache unless the person is especially anxious and upset.

Therapeutic Massage and Physical Therapy

Many physicians and hospitals have physical therapists on staff who can give deep therapeutic massages to help the back. The therapist can also give ultrasonic therapy (high-frequency sound waves), shortwave diathermy treatments (heat created by high-frequency electric currents), or hydrotherapy (therapy with water). These therapies are helpful to some people and not to others. Frequently, our patients report that these treatments are especially helpful in arthritis, bursitis of the shoulder, or tendinitis, where calcium forms along a tendon.

We find that ultrasound benefits are much greater when low-frequency treatments are used as opposed to high frequencies. Apparently the lower frequencies penetrate to a greater depth and so are more effective in relieving pain and stiffness. Ultrasound can also be used to drive corticosteroid through tissue to the site of injury, a more effective technique than giving corticosteroid by injection.

Electrical stimulation is a seldom-used but often effective pain reliever. The Egyptians used to place an electric fish from the Nile over a painful area. Today's technique uses a battery-powered electric current that a technician applies around a painful area or over the nerve going to it. The technique is reported to relieve pain in 80 percent of acute pain cases, but in only 25 percent of chronic pain cases. Electrical stimulation is very soothing and relaxing, and especially good for muscle spasms.

Therapeutic massage is very helpful for acute back pain that doesn't involve the nerves and for back pain that may occur after surgery. You can also have a therapist teach someone in your family to give you an at-home massage. Have them give you an all-body massage plus a gentle massage of the local painful area, using warm rubbing alcohol or witch hazel or a half-and-half mixture of the two. They should rub toward the heart, using fingertips, thumbs, knuckles, elbows—whatever feels good to you. They can knead gently, slowly pressing into the areas that are tender and holding the pressure for 7 to 10 seconds, or roll the skin gently between the fingers.

Massage reduces pain by helping to relax muscle spasms, relieve congestion, stimulate circulation, and relieve inflammation, but there may be one more reason that it helps pain—a mechanism that researchers call the "gate control theory." It goes like this: Pain impulses travel from the nerves to the spinal cord and then to the brain, which is where they are perceived as pain. Rubbing sends other impulses along the same nerves that can interfere with the pain impulses so that they don't get through the gate to the brain.

Note: Physical therapists often follow particular schools of approach. The McKenzie approach, for example, uses many extension exercises, as well as other techniques. The Feldenkrais method teaches the patient to improve control of body movements and to learn new patterns of more efficient movement. Rolfing involves manipulative procedures designed to reduce muscle dysfunction and tension. Others use myofascial release; that is, they work on the fascia, the tough connective tissue that surrounds muscles, bones, nerves, and body organs and that sometimes puts pressure on those structures, causing pain. Some use reflexology, pressing against certain points along the foot to produce pain relief in other parts of the body.

Trigger-Point Treatment

Many times when there is pain, the cause of that pain is somewhere else. A trigger point in the back might cause pain in the hip or arm. Or a trigger point in one part of the back could cause pain in another part of the back.

These highly irritable spots in muscles often are the cause of back pain, but unfortunately often go unrecognized.

Trigger points can occur in the neck, shoulders, back, and hip. They can be caused by frequent stress of a muscle, an acute strain, or muscle spasm.

Over the years, many people accumulate unsuspected trigger points. These may persist for years after an injury, and then may be activated by minor stresses such as periods of immobility, overstretching of muscles, or even chilling or fatigue. They also sometimes seem to be aggravated by tension, underactive thyroid, estrogen deficiency, chronic infection, anemia, low potassium and calcium levels, and vitamin B and C deficiencies.

Once the trigger points have formed, if untreated, the episodes of pain often increase both in intensity and frequency.

A trigger point can be identified by deep tenderness or pain in a hard-feeling band of muscle. Sometimes it can be worked out with massage. Or the skin can be cooled (but not the underlying muscle) with a coolant spray. The brief cooling of the skin has a reflex effect on the muscle that allows it to be stretched to its full length.

Massage or cooling of trigger points can be done at home by someone in your family after being shown the technique by a professional physical therapist. As in the therapeutic massage, they can use thumb, elbow, fingertips, or knuckles to find the sensitive points and press against them or on surrounding congested tissues. Have them let one area rest while doing other areas, and then return to areas that were especially painful.

When cold is applied, it is done by spraying a thin stream of a coolant in even sweeps over the trigger point, and then slowly sweeping it toward and over the area of referred pain. Sweeps are repeated in a steady rhythm of a few seconds on and a few seconds off, until all the skin over the areas is covered once or twice. While the coolant is being applied, the muscles are gently stretched to promote relaxation and increase the range of motion.

147

Sometimes a trigger point is injected with a local anesthetic, possibly combined with an anti-inflammatory, to break the circle of pain. This needs to be done with caution however; there might be an allergic reaction, so there should be emergency measures handy. Reactions are rare, but they can occur, and can include dangerous drops in blood pressure.

Trigger points can cause radiating pain to the back and down the legs or arms, just as a bulging disc can. In fact, many times a back pain sufferer with pain from a trigger point has been incorrectly diagnosed as having a bulging disc. But trigger points do not usually cause sensory loss, numbness, or weakness, as disc problems can.

If you have pain and want to determine whether you might have one trigger point or more, study the diagrams of some of the common trigger points and have someone push firmly on the various locations. If it is a trigger point causing pain, the pressure should produce local pain and may even make the

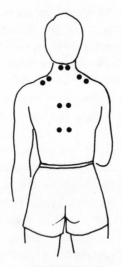

TRIGGER POINTS

muscle jump or twitch. Sometimes, if the point is pushed for several seconds, there will also be referred pain reproduced where you usually feel it, proving that this is at least one trouble spot.

Other Injections

In addition to injecting into a trigger point, injections are sometimes made directly into the area of a muscle spasm or into a joint such as the shoulder joint. Some patients also get relief from injections into scar tissue. Old scars, strangely, can sometimes set up pain patterns that go to deep tissues and show up as referred pain somewhere else in the body.

Occasionally steroids are injected directly into the spine area (called *epidural injection*). In one study, injections of hydrocortisone were given in patients with chronic spinal pain, and 57 percent had some relief of symptoms. Hydrocortisone combined with morphine is sometimes given before surgery. However, this technique was studied at the Institute in 600 cases, and it was found that there were many skin reactions and most people had only fair to no relief, so the technique was abandoned.

Sometimes there may be a nodule of fat on a back muscle that causes back pain and can be helped by injections. It can happen when a person strains the muscles of certain areas of the back, such as the sacroiliac, by lifting a heavy object improperly; then a small wedge of fat, the size of a thumb, can get displaced and cause pain. It may be treated by injecting the nodule with phenol combined with an anesthetic or an anti-inflammatory agent. The injections themselves cause pain for one to two days.

Traction

Some doctors consider traction helpful for back pain. The stretching is believed to widen the space between the vertebrae and so remove some pressure from the nerves. Other doctors consider the technique useless except as a device to keep the patient quiet and off his or her feet for a couple of days.

One version of stretching the spine is gravity lumbar reduction therapy, which is stretching using the weight of your body. The patient is placed in a chair or a standing frame and is fitted with a harness-vest to hold him or her off his or her feet.

Gravity traction is used primarily for patients with acute disc herniations. A typical maintenance program involves using the device 1 hour twice a day.

Dr. Charles Burton reports in the *Journal of Musculoskeletal Medicine* that at the Institute for Low Back Care in Minneapolis, doctors using the gravity reduction technique reported good to excellent results in 74 percent of patients hospitalized with acute disc herniation of less than six weeks' duration. However, the technique worked only in 32 percent of patients who had disc problems for longer times.

A less expensive and less drastic form of gravity traction is a bar put across a doorway. The patient hangs by the arms from the bar with feet held off the floor.

It is *not* recommended that you use inversion traction techniques. Upside-down suspension has been shown to alter seriously pressures inside the eyes and brain. Hanging from gravity boots and other inverted postures, for example, could be dangerous to patients with glaucoma and other eye disorders, could cause leaking of blood vessels in the eyes of persons with diabetes or sickle cell anemia, or could be dangerous in persons who have had past strokes or have weakened blood vessels in the brain.

Acupuncture

This technique has been around for thousands of years in China, has been available in France since 1934, and is now available in most areas of Europe, the Soviet Union, and the United States. It consists of inserting very thin needles—so thin they are really wires—into specific points on the skin. Chinese charts map from 385 to 1,000 points that relate to specific areas of the body. They apparently really do exist, because if you do electronic measurements, they show differences in the skin's electrical resistance at these various points.

When you have an acupuncture treatment, the thin wires are inserted into the points that relate to the area of pain that you have. There is no bleeding and, except for a tiny pricking or tingling sensation, no pain on insertion. After several needles are inserted, you may feel drowsy, and the area usually has a feeling of fullness and numbness, which the Chinese call *Da Chi*. The needles may be turned by hand or by a battery-powered instrument. A treatment takes from 10 minutes to 1 hour.

(Before having acupuncture, you should have a thorough examination to determine the cause of your pain. This is to prevent losing time from an accurate diagnosis of something that could be a warning sign of a serious disease.)

How effective is it in relieving pain? Many doctors claim dramatic relief in many patients even after other treatments have failed to relieve pain. Other doctors feel that the benefits are overrated. British scientists Drs. Charles Vincent and Phillip Richardson concluded after a review of the literature that 50 to 80 percent of patients with acute or chronic pain, including back pain, are helped at least temporarily by acupuncture. Other scientists have shown that acupuncture stimulates the production of pain-blocking chemicals and reduces inflammation. Dr. Miles Belgrade, neurologist and director of the pain clinic at Hennepin County Medical Center in Minnesota, says he finds acupuncture gives positive results in about 50 percent of the center's back patients.

An adequate trial for acupuncture is 6 to 10 treatments, 2 to 7 days apart. If you respond, your pain may disappear for days, months, or years; there is no way to tell. If you responded well and the pain later reappears, it usually is helpful to return for a booster treatment.

Acupuncturists should use presterilized, disposable needles. Acupuncture should not be used in heart attack patients or when there are acute infections.

Manipulation

Have you ever seen a dog do a morning stretch and spine extension, or watch a cat lie on its back and flex? That is a little bit of what manipulation is all about.

It's designed to rotate and bend the spine at different levels, to move the muscles and bones and joints in ways that relieve pressure and muscle spasm, and so relieve pain and stress and congestion and restore proper balance and function. Short muscles are stretched, tight muscles are relaxed. Sometimes you can actually hear a click or feel a sudden snapping of a joint as a certain manipulation is performed. It's similar to cracking your knuckles, but on a larger scale.

In one of the most common manipulations for low back pain, the doctor gently rotates your shoulders and hips in opposite directions while you are lying on your back or side. Putting traction on the head and neck to separate joints of the cervical spine is another frequently used technique and often helps to relieve neck pain.

At one time, only chiropractors and doctors of osteopathy used manipulation to treat low back pain and other problems, but now many other physicians and physical therapists are taking a look at manipulation and adopting it as another treatment technique in their practices.

Treatment by manipulation may be especially effective in early acute episodes of back pain. Let yourself relax as much as possible if you are having manipulation so that there will be less muscle tension around the joint being worked.

If manipulation is likely to involve pain or be particularly difficult, it should not be done.

Before any manipulation is performed, a thorough history and physical exam is necessary. You should not have spinal manipulation if you are pregnant or have a fever or if there is an inflammation or infection of the spine, a tumor, advanced osteoporosis, rheumatoid arthritis, disc bulging or rupture, a fracture, or a bleeding disorder.

Professional Machines for Back Strengthening

Excellent results are being obtained with several machines, such as the new Medex computerized lumbar extension machine for strengthening the lower back. Dr. Michael Pollock, director of the University of Florida's Center for Exercise Science, reports after testing the machine that using it can double lower back muscle strength in as few as 10 weeks.

Dr. Pollock explains that the lumbar muscles of the lower back are susceptible to injury because they are rarely used and are not trained by the usual exercise routines. The machine holds the pelvis immobile so that the buttocks and leg muscles cannot be used in back exercises so the smaller and weaker extensor muscles must do the work.

A person sits on a padded chair that restricts the motion of the torso and upper legs so that by pushing against resistance a person can specifically exercise the lumbar extensor back muscles. Exercises are done for about 10 minutes once a week for approximately 10 weeks.

Corsets and Bands

Your doctor may prescribe a fitted corset for temporary relief and stabilization of the back. Or you may be given a wide elastic abdominal binder to provide support. At GCOC we prefer not to use a corset unless a patient's abdomen is especially heavy. A potholder is not the answer, so if a corset is used, it should be only temporary; patients need to build up their own muscle strength for natural body support. As soon as your doctor says you can, start your back-strengthening exercises. Otherwise, you are likely to have further loss of muscle tone and stiffness of the spine.

For the pregnant woman who also has disc degeneration, a special supporting maternity corset may be helpful. A Japanese variation, centuries old, is the Iwata-Obi, made of approximately 5 yards of 8-inch-wide cotton cloth. The cloth is wrapped around the lower abdomen to provide support, especially during the last months of pregnancy.

Psychological Help

If your doctor's recommendations do not give you relief from your back pain, and you have completed our exercise program and still have no relief, you should be open-minded about seeing a mental health professional to investigate the possibility of emotional factors and to get help for them. Often there are hidden emotional factors that bother us more than we realize.

However, remember that just because the doctor cannot find a cause for your back pain does not mean that it is all in your mind. It could be that the cause of the pain has not yet been found. Many people believe that if a pain patient is depressed, it is the depression that is causing the pain. Not necessarily true. It can be the other way around. The chronic pain may *create* anxiety and depression. When your back hurts all the time, it can bring on depression, anxiety, frustration and fatigue, and it can make it hard to work productively and to live a happy life.

Be assured that just because you might need some help emotionally doesn't mean that you are faking your pain, or imagining it. Your pain is real, but it is perhaps being increased by some hidden tensions and anxieties or other problems. Stress, for example, may be causing muscle tension that aggravates a strained back muscle.

If depression is a problem, you might be helped by a medication to help depression.

For stress, there are a number of psychological techniques that might prove beneficial, such as biofeedback, relaxation techniques, group therapy, and others. GCOC finds biofeedback especially helpful in many patients.

Another effective technique used by psychologists, called neurolinguistic programming (NLP), is to place yourself mentally back to a time and place before you had pain and focus on every detail. Create the view, the sounds, and the smells, and let yourself feel as you did then and have the posture that you did then. Enlarge those feelings and imprint the pictures and feelings into your body language.

A professional interested in emotional factors might also teach you to use a healing phrase, a positive affirmation of health, such as "I am getting healthier and feeling better and stronger and more energetic every day."

If you have chronic pain, the National Chronic Pain Outreach Association suggests that, in addition to an exercise program and relaxation techniques, you do the following:

- Avoid isolation; join a pain support group.
- Keep active and occupied with activities that are meaningful to you. (Pace yourself; don't overdo or underdo.)
- Decide what's most important to you, set realistic goals, and focus your energies toward these goals.

- Educate yourself about your condition and appropriate treatment options and explore different treatment methods, giving each a fair chance.
- Cultivate a positive attitude (negative thinking increases pain).
- Focus on what you *can* do, not on what you can't do.

Religious faith can also enhance treatment. At a special session on the role of faith in the treatment of patients with back pain at the annual meeting of the American Back Society, Dr. William H. Kirkaldy-Willis told participants that in his experience, visualization and imagery can be used for back pain patients just as it is now being used for cancer patients. The patient makes a picture in his mind of the problem and then visualizes recovery actually taking place. Kirkaldy-Willis and other back specialists at the meeting encouraged patients to add prayer—by themselves and with others—to their other treatments.

When Pain Doesn't Go Away

Sometimes back pain doesn't seem to respond to any ordinary treatments, not even to surgery. The pain just goes on and on no matter what treatments are undertaken.

But there are still things that can be tried, techniques such as biofeedback, hypnosis, and ways of blocking nerve impulses that are proving effective for pain control when other methods have failed.

If your back is still painful after you have tried exercises and other programs recommended by your physician, you may want to consider one or more of the following. Best results are often obtained with a combination of two procedures.

Biofeedback
Biofeedback is a technique designed to teach you to control body functions and help you to control pain. You learn how to

manipulate your muscle tension or skin temperature or other function by watching its measurement on a screen and getting the feel of what makes it go up or down. Biofeedback has been shown to be helpful in counteracting back pain, fighting stress, and treating such things as headache, high blood pressure, insomnia, heart arrhythmias, and speech problems.

Hypnosis

If you decide to use hypnosis, you should be taught by a professional; then you can do it at home yourself if you wish. Commercial tapes are also available. Hypnosis does not cure the source of the pain, but it makes you feel it less.

After becoming relaxed, you give yourself a specific message. Use positive terms. (Don't say "I'm not going to hurt," but tell yourself something that you *are* going to do, such as "I am going to float the pain away," or "I am going to turn down the volume of the pain like the volume on the radio, so I can barely feel it anymore.")

Caution: Don't overdo activity just because you can't feel the pain. Let your back muscles slowly return to normal.

TENS

Transcutaneous electrical nerve stimulation (TENS) is the primary method of pain control at GCOC. It uses an instrument that puts out low electric current to stimulate the skin at traditional acupuncture sites. By electrically scrambling the pain signal in the nerve fibers, the TENS blocks discomfort before it reaches the brain. A small battery-powered stimulator is worn by the patient, and the patient is taught to turn the TENS on as needed. The amplitude and frequency of the impulses can be controlled by two dials as desired, according to what works best for the pain. A strong tingling sensation is felt.

Sometimes TENS treatment is combined with traditional acupuncture. It is an excellent technique to prevent the chronic pain sufferer from becoming addicted to pain drugs.

At GCOC we pioneered the use of TENS in patients in the recovery room to eliminate pain after surgery.

Implants

Just as TENS units can be used on the skin to give electric stimulation, a special unit can be permanently implanted to give stimulation and deaden pain on command. The epidural electrical stimulation device (EES) was approved by the Food and Drug Administration (FDA) in 1986. It is implanted in or near the spinal cord, with wires running under the skin to a tiny radio receiver just under the skin on the chest. When needed, the patient activates the system with a battery-operated transmitter strapped to the waist. Impulses block pain signals from going to the brain. You can wear the device for as many hours as needed, and then untape it when desired.

Pain Clinics

Specialized pain clinics have been established in a number of medical centers to deal with chronic pain. They usually use all of the techniques just outlined plus dietary instruction, vitamin therapy, exercises, psychological counseling, stress management, treatment of depression, physical therapy, and drug withdrawal.

Most of the centers incorporate both standard treatments and newer approaches. The goal: to eliminate or reduce pain significantly, or, if that's impossible, to help the patient learn to cope with the disability, to be free of drugs, and to return to a more normal, productive life.

A major goal of a pain center is to change the attitudes of patients so that they can get on with their lives. It is so easy to slip into the habit of using pain as a focus of one's life, to avoid work or to get attention and sympathy by letting people know how much you bravely suffer. Sometimes, without realizing it, patients let their lives get built around their pain, and they need help in breaking the habit.

How to Resume Activity Following a Back Problem

It is important to get back to work as quickly as you physically can without danger to your back. The more weeks that go by, the less probability of your returning to work with full activity. Latest studies show that very few people who have been out of work with back pain for six months or more ever return.

We recommend the following program:

- Give your back as much rest as it seems to need; then resume activities gradually and cautiously. Avoid *strenuous* activity—it can bring the problem back and delay recovery.
- Start gentle stretching exercises and back-building exercises.
- Practice good posture rules on driving and lifting, as outlined in other sections of this book.
- Avoid fatigue.
- Avoid lifting of any kind. Baby yourself for a few weeks, and let someone else do all the lifting and heavy work.

But, *do* become active again. Be careful that you don't get caught in that vicious cycle: pain making you inactive, inactivity causing physical deconditioning, poor condition causing more pain, and on and on. Attitude—not letting yourself feel disabled—can be one of the most significant factors in a patient's progress. The earlier you become active again, the more likely you will get back to completely normal activity.

In the next chapter we will talk about medicines that might be useful for back pain. However, we urge you to remember that although the treatments in this chapter and the medicines in the next chapter are often helpful, you need to think not only in terms of eliminating pain, but also about going beyond pain relief to increasing function and preventing further back problems. It could be a serious mistake to assume you are well just because your pain has gone away. You need to get to the *cause* of your problem and to strengthen your back muscles. For that, you still need to do the exercises and the other phases of the total program.

It is also important that you stay in charge of your back. Work with your doctor or other professionals, but do not turn your back over to their control or to drugs. You are in charge; you are responsible for doing what is necessary to make your back better.

CHAPTER TWELVE

Painkillers, Muscle Spasm Drugs, and Other Medicines You Should Know About

Most back sufferers can be helped with the program of new body mechanics (Chapter 5) plus the exercise program (Chapter 4) with occasional use of the instant techniques for relief (Chapter 3) and various nondrug treatments. These methods should be your first line of defense. Indeed, at their most recent conference on the management of pain, the National Institutes of Health stressed the recent advances and increasing role of nondrug treatment of pain and encouraged its use. However, there are some people who may need medication if these techniques are not enough.

Pain medications have been used through the ages. The Babylonians used herbs for pain relief as far back as 2250 B.C.; the Egyptians recorded the use of opium in 1550 B.C.; the Chinese used various herbs to treat pain, including the poppy and its derivative, opium.

Most of the medicines used today to treat the back are prescribed either to ease pain, to fight inflammation, or to relax muscle spasm. They can come in the form of pills, injections, or applications to the skin.

In this chapter we will tell you about the medicines that you are the most likely to encounter.

But Before You Use Any Medicine

Remember that a treatment that works for one person may not help another. Doses vary according to a person's rate of metabolism, variation in age and body size, and other factors. If you need a pill, it should be prescribed by your physician specifically to treat your particular problem and circumstances, to best fit your special needs.

Don't take pills without consulting a physician. Don't take pills if you don't really need them. Don't take them for a longer time or in larger doses than you have been instructed. Get off them as soon as you can.

This is especially true of painkillers. Using a painkiller makes sense if you can't sleep because of pain, or if you take it for a short time while your doctor investigates the source of your problem and treats it. But find the cause of your back pain and work to correct it rather than use pain pills on a long-term basis.

If you are pregnant, you should not take *any* pain medicine, even if you have severe back pain. Many medicines, even something as simple as aspirin, are transmitted to the developing fetus, and you never know which of them, even in small doses, could cause damage to your developing baby.

Also remember to keep all pill bottles out of the reach of children. Painkillers or other back medicines may be powerful enough to kill a child if taken in quantity.

Linaments, Lotions, Ointments, and Balms

The scientific terminology is *topical medicines*—medicines that you apply locally to the skin.

Many of them, such as Ben-Gay, Icy Hot, Tiger Balm, and oil of wintergreen, are available over the counter and work by stimulating the circulation of blood to the affected area and producing heat. They help low back pain that does not have radiating pain down the arm or leg.

If you use them, follow a few precautions: Don't use a heating pad when you use a skin application; and don't cover the area with anything other than a normal fabric; either one could injure the skin.

Note on DMSO. Dimethyl sulfoxide, or DMSO, is a controversial "alternative" medication that is patted on painful muscles and joints. Those who use it report that it reduces pain and increases joint mobility in pulled muscles, strains, and osteoarthritis. DMSO is also reported to be effective for reducing pain and swelling in bursitis, tendinitis, and sprains and stimulates healing of open wounds, burns, and skin ulcers, and sometimes relieves the pain of shingles and bedsores. The GCOC Institute has not used it, but some of our patients have. You will have to test its effectiveness yourself.

DMSO has the unique property of being absorbed almost instantly through the skin to the bloodstream, thus going quickly throughout the body. Do not mix other medications or ointments with DMSO since it will carry them through the skin.

Not many physicians use DMSO in the United States, but it is available in most health food stores in the United States and is used frequently by veterinarians in the United States to treat animals and by physicians in Europe. To use it, you simply dab it on the skin with cotton, and then stay away from friends—it works well but smells terrible. Some physicians are using it experimentally as a base to carry topical steroids quickly into deep tissue to help various back problems.

If You Use Aspirin

One or two tablets of aspirin every 4 to 6 hours plus bedrest is the advice most commonly recommended for the relief of back pain. Aspirin relieves pain, reduces fever and inflammation, and is cheap, but it can cause side effects, acting as an anticlotting agent and sometimes causing stomach bleeding or aggravation of ulcers. (Use a buffered kind.) Acetaminophen (Tylenol) will work against pain, but it does not relieve stiffness or tissue inflammation.

If taken in large amounts over long periods, aspirin can cause ringing in the ears and dizziness or even contribute to deafness. If you are taking aspirin regularly and have one or more of these symptoms, stop taking the aspirin and call your doctor.

Aspirin can also sometimes cause hypoglycemia (a fall in blood sugar), which in turn can be the cause of other symptoms, including fatigue, irritability, and tension.

If you take aspirin, always take it with a full glass of water, to prevent stomach irritation. Do *not* take aspirin (or products like Alka-Seltzer that contain aspirin) if you have stomach distress or if you have an ulcer. Do *not* take aspirin or products containing aspirin if you are pregnant. Do *not* mix aspirin with beer, wine, or liquor (the mixing increases stomach irritation). Do *not* take aspirin if you are taking other medicine for pain, medicine for thinning the blood, or medicine for diabetes.

If you use a lot of aspirin, take vitamin C supplements regularly since aspirin depletes vitamin C from the body.

If you're allergic to aspirin, you should avoid medications that contain aspirinlike ingredients. (Watch for the word *salicylate* on the label.)

Don't take aspirin for several weeks prior to elective surgery, unless your doctor specifically recommends it, since it will increase bleeding.

Children and young adults, ages 2 to 20, should *not* take aspirin for backaches, especially if they have chicken pox or any flulike symptoms. It can cause Reye's syndrome, a rare but potentially fatal condition.

Codeine and Morphine

If pain is so severe you cannot rest, your doctor may give you codeine or aspirin and codeine together. Codeine belongs in the class of opiates (as does morphine). Dizziness, drowsiness, fatigue, a flushed face, and difficulty in urinating often occur as side effects. Constipation sometimes occurs.

If your pain is severe and your doctor prescribes codeine, take it only when needed, since codeine products can sometimes be addictive. They also can interact with other drugs, such as sleeping pills, antidepressants, and tranquilizers, to produce an increased sedative effect.

The vast majority of patients can be helped with the other treatments we have described, but when these fail, then for those few patients who still have pain, it may be necessary to use these stronger painkillers. Pain patients should not have to suffer needless agony.

In a recent issue of *Scientific American*, Dr. Ronald Melzack, an internationally known pain scientist and research director of the Pain Clinic of Montreal General Hospital in Canada, cited two studies of more than 10,000 patients each that showed that, contrary to popular belief, narcotics taken solely for pain are not usually addictive. The typical pattern, he said, is that patients may develop some tolerance at first and need some increased dosage, but that this stabilizes, with little further tolerance developing.

The National Institutes of Health conference on pain that we mentioned earlier reported that children may be the main group especially being undertreated. There have been many shocking reports of children not being given pain medication when they are in pain, even after surgery.

Strong painkillers should not be used routinely, but when there is severe pain, there is a place for them, particularly for temporary relief while a treatment plan is being worked out. If your doctor does prescribe a painkiller, you must be careful to control your physical activity so that you do not unknowingly cause further injury.

Muscle Relaxants

Muscle relaxant medicines occasionally can be effective in helping to break the cycle of muscle spasm and thus alleviate pain, but they should only be used if there are spasms and if the patient stays in bed, and only for two to three weeks at most. Try the nondrug ways discussed in earlier chapters. Many relaxants produce drowsiness, so don't drive or operate dangerous equipment if you take them.

Usually a muscle spasm is secondary to a primary problem, and when the primary problem is diagnosed and treated, the spasm will usually subside.

Tranquilizers and Antidepressants

We do not recommend that patients use tranquilizers for pain— unless the pain is accompanied by a lot of tension and anxiety, or if the patient has long-standing pain resulting in anxiety or depression.

If it is decided that a tranquilizer or antidepressant is necessary, it should be chosen carefully by a physician who is familiar with the various side effects, because all tranquilizers and antidepressants are not alike. For example, some tranquilizers also have muscle relaxant properties. Other tranquilizers can increase the depression that frequently accompanies back pain and so would not be desirable to use.

Some antidepressants have been shown to increase the perception of pain; others do not. Some, such as Elavil and Prozac, can also help counteract back pain.

These are finely tuned decisions to be made by a knowledgeable physician.

If an antidepressant is used, it should be started at a low dosage for one week, increasing the dosage the following week. When it is stopped, the dosage should be lowered gradually to prevent the possibility of depression.

But these drugs are not going to cure your back pain. They can sometimes be helpful, and should be used as needed, but only temporarily. The *cause* of your back pain should be found and treated.

Corticosteroids

Corticosteroids are excellent anti-inflammatory agents and are frequently prescribed for arthritis and other inflammatory conditions such as bursitis. They are manufactured drugs that closely resemble cortisone, a natural hormone produced by the body. They sometimes, but not always, will help back pain due to inflammation. Steroids may be taken orally or injected directly into an inflamed joint. There are frequent side effects, including irritability of the digestive tract, weight gain, depletion of calcium, osteoporosis, water retention, cataracts, and decreased immune mechanisms.

If you have ever had tuberculosis, diabetes, or ulcers, you should not be given any cortisone or cortisone products.

If you develop a persistent backache when you have been taking any corticosteroid product over a long period, contact your doctor. There is a chance that you are developing osteoporosis, often a side effect to taking steroid drugs. Our Institute doctors recommend that calcium routinely be given right from the beginning with cortisone to *prevent* the bone changes and backache from occurring and that hormone levels be carefully monitored.

Be sure when your doctor has you stop taking cortisone that he or she reduces the dosage slowly, not all at once to reduce side effects. Follow the schedule exactly, even if it seems complicated.

The NSAID Drugs

More than 50 million prescriptions for nonsteroidal anti-inflammatory drugs (NSAIDs) are written in the United States per year, and they are now available over the counter as well as by prescription. They bring about pain relief by inhibiting the production of prostaglandin hormones that carry pain impulses to the brain. However, the NSAIDs are known to cause injury to the linings of the stomach and small intestine, sometimes causing ulcers, especially in older patients. In fact, a number of studies have shown a possible association between these drugs and deaths in older people from fatal internal bleeding. The NSAIDs are also known to restrict blood flow to the kidneys and thus can cause kidney failure, even in patients who have only mild kidney problems. A study at Johns Hopkins School of Medicine showed that even an over-the-counter strength of some NSAIDs could cause kidney failure in high-risk people within several days. If you on occasion take one or two tablets a day, there is no reason to worry, experts say, but if your doctor puts you on NSAIDs for a long period, you should be tested regularly for osteoporosis or changes in kidney function.

Ibuprofen is one form of NSAID. Some strengths are available only by prescription and are indicated for serious pain and only under a physician's care. Over-the-counter forms—Motrin IB, Advil, Medipren, and Nuprin—are for temporary relief of minor aches, pain, and fever due to headaches, toothaches, backache, arthritis pain, or menstrual cramps.

Ibuprofen is generally considered more effective for back pain than are aspirin or regular-strength Tylenol tablets, and it doesn't irritate the stomach the way aspirin can. However, even with over-the-counter forms of ibuprofen, you should never take more than six tablets in 24 hours.

Sulindac is an NSAID that has been shown to be effective in the treatment of most kinds of arthritis, including rheumatoid arthritis, osteoarthritis, gout, and ankylosing spondylitis. It is about as effective as eight aspirins per day and is also less irritating to the stomach.

Another NSAID is flurbiprofen, used mostly for relieving pain and inflammation in rheumatoid arthritis and osteoarthritis. Clinical trials have shown it to be effective at lower doses than ibuprofen and aspirin, sometimes improving mobility in rheumatoid arthritis in as little as a week. Side effects occur only about half as often as with indomethacin and aspirin, but it still should be used with caution in patients with current or past kidney or liver problems. Common side effects are ulcers, vision problems, and fluid retention.

Indomethacin (Indocin), another NSAID drug, is beneficial to about 50 percent of patients with rheumatoid arthritis. It is not usually used in osteoarthritis, except for osteoarthritis of the hip, for which it often provides dramatic relief. It is also effective in the treatment of ankylosing spondylitis and gout. Because of its many side effects, the doctors at the Institute do not recommend it for simple back pain. Some patients experience nausea or headache, but this goes away with continued use. Indomethacin can irritate the stomach and so should be taken immediately after meals. Long use may cause eye problems or anemia, so if you take it on a long-term basis, you should have an eye examination by an ophthalmologist every 6 to 12 months and a blood test. Stop taking it if you develop headaches or blurred vision.

A caution to remember with any NSAID is that these drugs lower fevers, so that if you contract an infection, you might not realize its seriousness, since you might not have the fever that would ordinarily occur.

No NSAID should be used in children, pregnant women, nursing mothers, patients with ulcers, or patients allergic to aspirin. Mental alertness may be reduced by some of them, so do not drive or use dangerous tools. When back pain goes away, call your doctor so that he can tell you how to taper off the drug.

Other Medicines You Should Know About

Colchicine

This gout medicine is sometimes used in back patients with good results. It should be taken with food to lessen stomach irritation, nausea, and diarrhea.

Penicillamine

This medication is sometimes used in arthritis, but it is rarely used for simple backache. It appears to provide slow but long-term benefits in some patients, but it has a great many side effects. Current recommendations are that patients take this medication only if they do not respond to other treatment, and they should have frequent blood and urine tests to monitor for trouble.

This medicine should only be started at a very low level and be built up slowly. Typical side effects that may sometimes occur include nausea, skin rash, mouth sores, blood disorders, and kidney damage.

Gold Compounds

Gold pills are reported to take effect in about five weeks

(gold injections take about three months) with reduction of joint pain, swelling, and stiffness. But there are severe side effects, and this medicine is now seldom used.

Phenylbutazone

This drug, also known as Butazolidin, is sometimes used to treat ankylosing spondylitis, but because there often are side effects, it should be used at the lowest possible dosage and patients using it should have frequent blood counts. It is also effective in osteoarthritis, gout, and bursitis. It should be taken with meals or milk and should be accompanied by antacid therapy. It should not be taken with any blood-thinning drugs and should only be used with caution in heart patients.

Superoxide Dismutase

S.O.D. is an anti-inflammatory drug used for arthritis and inflammations. Although controversial, it appears to have benefit in rheumatoid arthritis, osteoarthritis, spondylosis and disc disease.

Gerovital

For the past 20 years, thousands of patients have gone to clinics in Europe to receive treatments with a controversial Romanian drug called Gerovital. It is a mixture of procaine (Novocain) and several other substances that the developer of the drug claims is effective in treating depression and memory loss as well as arthritis and osteoporosis.

There are two forms of the drug: KH-3, developed in West Germany, and Gerovital H-3, developed by Dr. Ana Aslan of Romania. Both drugs were being tested in the United States as this book went to press. Simple procaine without the various additions found in these formulas seems to not have the effect of the combination drugs.

Possible Side Effects to Be Alert for with Any Drug

Call your doctor if you are taking medicine and any of the following signs of a reaction occur:

- Dizziness
- Nausea or vomiting
- Wheezing or shortness of breath
- Inflammation of the eyelids or reddening of the eyes
- Skin rash, itching, or hives
- Blood in the urine or stool
- Diarrhea
- An agitated or upset emotional state
- Headache
- Ringing in the ears

The Safe Way to Use Medications for Back Pain

Always tell a new physician of any past drug reaction, even if it was mild. The next reaction may be more severe, and indeed could be life threatening.

Tell your physician of *any* medicine you are taking—whether it's an over-the-counter pill or a prescription from another physician, even if it's something as simple as aspirin or sleeping pills. There may be possible interactions between the pills that this doctor would give you and the other pills you are taking. For example, aspirin can counteract the action of gout pills and can increase the action of anticoagulants. Some arthritis medicines can decrease the effectiveness of birth control pills. If you mix some arthritis medications such as indomethacin with an anticoagulant such as Coumadin, blood thinning can be increased so much that there is danger of internal hemorrhaging.

Tell your doctor if you use drugs, or are a heavy drinker, or if you smoke cigarettes. Alcohol taken with a barbiturate could kill you. Alcohol taken with aspirin can cause stomach bleeding.

Tell your doctor if you have some kind of chronic problem such as epilepsy, an eye disorder, heart trouble, an ulcer, diabetes, asthma, emphysema, kidney trouble, or liver disease. These conditions could necessitate changes in dosages or make you more vulnerable to certain side effects. For example if you are diabetic, your insulin could be neutralized by aspirin and some other arthritis medicines.

When your doctor prescribes a drug, ask the name of the drug and what it is supposed to do. Make sure you understand how and when it should be taken, when it should not be taken, and what side effects you should be especially alert for. Ask what precautions should be observed while taking the medicine, such as avoiding driving or operating machinery because the medicine makes you drowsy or avoiding certain foods or drinks. Know whether the prescription should be refilled or not. Ask when you should report back to the doctor.

Make sure your medicines are labeled as to their contents so that you know exactly what the medication is. Do not accept an unknown remedy without explanation. To be an intelligent patient, you need to know what you are taking, and why. This information is also valuable if you change physicians.

Read the label. Follow all instructions and warnings. Never exceed the listed maximum dosage.

Don't change dosages or stop taking the medicine without consulting your doctor. If you are having side effects or are otherwise dissatisfied with the medication, call and ask for advice. There are many things that can be done. For example, some people have more tolerance for pain in the morning than in the evening, so your doctor may be able to lessen your dosage in the morning.

Always discard medicines on their expiration date and

throw away any medicine that has turned color, has congealed, has started to crumble, or smells like vinegar, or if you're not sure what it is.

Do not use any medicine for your back without your doctor's advice and a clear understanding of how long you should use the medicine, and be sure that any medicine that is prescribed for you on a long-term basis is periodically evaluated by your doctor and not automatically continued.

Remember: any medicine you take can harm your body. Pain medication, tranquilizers, and antidepressants can all be supporting steps that can be used to help a patient, but no medication is a substitute for an accurate diagnosis and a specific treatment. The sooner a diagnosis is reached and proper treatment started, the better the results you will have.

CHAPTER THIRTEEN

The Most Common Causes of Lingering Back Pain and What to Do About Them

Many cases of back pain are short-term problems: you overworked in the garden, you shoveled snow too vigorously, you hurt your back in an accident; or your back pain may be due mostly to a sedentary life, easily correctable with our exercise program. But many other cases are due to a body disorder that is long term, which means your back problem is chronic and not so easily dealt with.

In this chapter we will deal with arthritis, osteoporosis, slipped disc and other problems that are the most common causes of lingering chronic back pain.

Arthritis—The Disease of Many Faces

There are many different kinds of arthritis, and they vary greatly in severity from one person to another. In addition, many things mimic arthritis. So if you think you have arthritis, it is important for you to see a doctor to find out if you really have arthritis or something else and to find the appropriate treatment.

175

Remember, as in any disorder, but especially in arthritis conditions: Some treatments work for some people and not for others; and some work at one stage of the disease and not at other stages.

The following are the most common types of arthritis that can affect the back.

Rheumatoid Arthritis.   This arthritis can occur at any age, from childhood to old age. Women are affected two to three times more often than men are. The condition usually begins with swelling of the joints of the fingers and toes; sometimes there also is pain, numbness, or tingling. As the disease progresses, it may spread to other joints—the wrists, elbows, knees, shoulders, hips, and spine. There is often muscle stiffness, especially in the morning or after periods of inactivity. It usually becomes worse with time. Symptoms seem to come and go—there are remissions, then recurrences of symptoms, so that neither the patient nor the doctor can predict the pattern of the disease. During active attacks, there is often fever.

Juvenile rheumatoid arthritis   (also known as Still's disease). This especially affects children under age 5 and usually involves the neck. See a doctor if your child shows a reluctance to crawl or walk or cries when limbs are moved. Other symptoms may include fever, rash, and involvement of the wrist or finger joints as well as the neck. There may be only one occurrence, or it may be persistent.

Ankylosing Spondylitis   (Marie-Strumpell's disease). Once called rheumatoid spondylitis, this is a progressive inflammatory form of arthritis that sometimes attacks the back. It generally affects persons between ages 20 and 40, although it can begin as early as age 10. Blacks in Africa seldom get it; North American Indians frequently do. The onset may be slow or sudden. There is early-morning pain and stiffness, often lasting several hours, then returning in the evening. As the disease progresses, there is increasing stiffness, especially of the lower back and sacroiliac joints, usually with pain in the buttocks and thighs.

Sometimes muscle spasms and back pain may be so severe that bending over is the only way to relieve it. Strangely, it is often associated with discomfort of the eyes and with ulcerative colitis (a kind of ulcer of the lower intestine that promotes diarrhea). Recent research at the University of Texas Southwestern Medical Center and the Howard Hughes Medical Institute indicates that both lowered immunity and ankylosing spondylitis are linked together to the same inherited gene.

Osteoarthritis. There is no fever or inflammation with osteoarthritis. It usually occurs after age 50, but can appear earlier. Bony growths form at the edges of joints, making them swollen and knobby. It can occur in the finger joints or in the hip, neck, knees, and back. Symptoms are especially common in people who have engaged in years of heavy labor or are overweight. When pain first appears, the person may walk stiffly and awkwardly, with one foot turned out. As the disease progresses, pain increases, and movement may become limited. On the other hand, many people show signs of osteoarthritis on X ray, but never have symptoms.

Arthritis Treatments

Because the forms of arthritis differ from patient to patient, each person's needs and treatment program will vary. Still, treatment for all forms usually involves several common elements— exercise, heat, physical therapy, and loss of excessive weight.

When a joint is inflamed, the joint should be rested and no weight should be put on it. In fact, in a severe attack of rheumatoid arthritis, complete bedrest is recommended; but bedrest usually is not needed for osteoarthritis.

Many arthritis patients get progressively weaker because they do not move enough. And if they reduce their physical activity, which only rarely is necessary, their poor condition can get even worse. Plenty of exercise is essential to build up muscle strength and flexibility of joints (except during the times joints are inflamed). Many arthritis patients at the GCOC Institute claim relief from pain for the first time after taking up the exercise program. Exercises that increase the range of motion are especially good in relieving problems of stiffness. Actress Debbie Reynolds is a good example of the value of exercise. Reynolds says she suffers from arthritis in her knees and back and is helped by walking on a treadmill in her home while watching old movies on television.

However, keep in mind the "Two-Hour Pain Rule": Any exercise that causes pain that lasts for more than two hours should be reduced.

Heat treatments often help arthritis. Hot tub baths, hot moist towels, heat lamps, heating pads, paraffin baths, or exercises in a warm-water pool can all be helpful. On the other hand, for some reason, some people find cold compresses or ice packs work better. Try both for yourself. Some people are helped by a change to a hot, dry climate.

Regular massage and physiotherapy, and sometimes gentle manipulation done periodically, can help also. A new experimental treatment, low-energy laser therapy, has been used in Europe and Japan to reduce pain and inflammation in patients with rheumatoid arthritis. In the United States, it is being studied at the Mayo Clinic.

Various studies have reported benefit to arthritis patients from increased amounts of calcium, magnesium, folic acid (especially in some patients with rheumatoid arthritis), niacin, vitamin D, vitamin E, and zinc. In one study patients with chronic rheumatoid arthritis given zinc supplements three times daily had less joint tenderness, swelling, and stiffness. (See Chapter 9 for other dietary advice.)

Maintaining normal weight is very important. If you are obese, you are putting a great strain on your joints. You will be much better off if you lose the weight.

Medications usually used for arthritis include aspirin, nonsteroidal anti-inflammatory drugs (NSAIDs), and corticosteroids; and if none of these works, the doctor may try other drugs.

And this may surprise you—investigators have found that some patients who have arthritislike symptoms really have a mild form of lead poisoning. If this is a problem, lead can be eliminated from your body with certain mineral supplements such as zinc, calcium, and magnesium in the proper ratios (do it through a doctor knowledgeable in nutrition), or if the condition is severe, by having slow intravenous injections of a chemical called EDTA that eliminates the lead (called chelation).

Gout

Gout usually attacks a big toe, but it can also occur in the spine or hip joint. It is caused by a deposit of urate crystals in the joint.

Treatment is with colchicine, indomethacin, or phenylbutazone. If the condition is chronic, the patient should not eat peanuts, organ meats such as kidneys and liver, and other foods with high uric acid content.

Fibrositis

Also called fibromyalgia or fibromyositis, this is a strange disorder that often mimics arthritis with symptoms of all-over achiness, pains, and stiffness, often of many joints, and characterized by nonrestorative sleep (with the sufferer waking up in the morning after a night's sleep still tired). Those afflicted are more sensitive to pain in the morning than they are in the evening, and have malaise—they just don't feel good. "Fibrositis" refers to local "tender points," sometimes felt with the fingers as irregular places on the muscle surface. The condition is often misdiagnosed as arthritis. Doctors don't really know what causes it.

Sleep researchers have found that people who have this set of symptoms have a different sleep wave pattern, with brain waves that are a mixture of sleep waves and waking waves, as though they were awake and asleep at the same time (called alpha-delta sleep).

Fibrositis/fibromylagia can occur in both adults and children.

The administration of low dosages of the antidepressant Elavil (10–25 mg) often helps to clear up the problem. This is apparently not because such patients are depressed, but because Elavil changes brain chemistry, and this somehow helps the sleep-wake "switch" to be thrown more firmly toward sleep, rather than being stuck in the middle.

In addition to a low dose of Elavil, nonjarring exercise, such as walking, swimming, or low-impact aerobics is recommended.

Paget's Disease

This disease of the bone, also called *osteitis deformans*, is often associated with osteoarthritis. The disease may start in middle age, or not become apparent until age 60 or later. In most patients there are no symptoms; the diagnosis is made by discovery on routine X ray, and no treatment is necessary.

Sometimes the disorder is more active, however, in which case the bones may weaken, and there may be easy fracturing. For patients with the more active form of Paget's, there now are several effective agents for relieving symptoms. Vitamin C and calcitonin, for example, have been shown to give some relief of pain.

Reiter's Syndrome

The cause of Reiter's syndrome is unknown, but it often follows an intestinal or genitourinary infection.

Symptoms include a strange three-way combination: inflammation of the urethra, inflammation of the membrane of the eye or other mucous membranes, *plus* arthritis, including arthritis of the spine. It can occur at any age, even in children, but is most common between the ages of 20 and 40. There seems to be a hereditary tendency to develop the disease. The three-way combination of symptoms can occur at the same time or within a few days or weeks of each other. Joint pain may occur in the extremities, especially the feet, or appear as low back pain, and usually lasts about three months or longer.

Aspirin and other anti-inflammatory drugs are the usual treatment.

Osteoporosis

In osteoporosis, a person's bones become less dense and the total amount of bone also decreases. The condition can occur in both men or women, occurring most often in women after menopause or after surgical removal of the ovaries. In fact, it occurs more commonly in women than breast cancer, heart attacks, diabetes, or arthritis.

Osteoporosis may result from a lack of calcium in the diet or from the body not being able to absorb calcium, or it may occur with prolonged treatment with corticosteroids. It is made worse by insufficient physical activity or weight-bearing exercise. (Bone loss is accelerated in astronauts in space when there is no gravity acting on their bones.) Often several of these factors occur together.

You are at greater risk of getting osteoporosis if you are thin, Caucasian or Asian (blacks have stronger bones and therefore less osteoporosis), have a close relative with osteoporosis, smoke, or consume excessive amounts of alcohol or caffeine. (One study found that the people who were 55 and drank 5 pints of beer a day had bone tissues that looked like that found in a 75-year-old person with osteoporosis.) It also increases your risk if you are on long-term treatment with antiseizure medication, cortisone, or aluminum-containing antacids.

Symptoms may start gradually, with periods of pain in the back, or symptoms thought to be arthritis followed by periods of improvement. Later there may be humping of the back and rounded shoulders—"dowager's hump"—so often seen in older people. Bone fractures may occur after what seems like the mildest bump. A person can crack a rib by turning in bed. Or bones can snap simply from carrying too much body weight. In fact, older people who have fallen and broken a hip often have actually had a hip bone break spontaneously from a slight stress, *after* which they fall because of the broken hip. Sometimes vertebrae of the spine may collapse or fracture. Recent estimates are that osteoporosis is responsible for nearly ½ million fractures every year.

Prevention. To help prevent osteoporosis you should start with a program as early as possible, especially if there is a history of osteoporosis in your family. Adolescents and young adults should have regular exercise and sufficient calcium intake. This, researchers believe, will ensure that bones reach peak density by the time the person reaches his or her thirties and thus help to protect against osteoporosis later. The exercise/calcium program should continue through your lifetime.

Make an effort to be active and get plenty of regular exercise, especially weight-bearing exercise (when you're in a standing position and your bones are supporting your body weight, as in walking, cross-country skiing, dancing), the best for strengthening bones. Do not let yourself become totally immobilized. Even if you have a chronic disease or are disabled, ask your doctor how you can exercise to some degree.

Eat a well-balanced diet with plenty of calcium. Both men and women should take calcium supplements. (Although it's not known for sure that more calcium now will prevent bone loss later, researchers believe that the evidence is still in favor of it.) Keep phosphorus intake low since high phosphorus ingestion is believed to add to bone loss. (Carbonated soft drinks and meat contain much phosphorus.)

Do not smoke, and keep alcohol to a minimum. The combination of smoking and drinking can increase your risk of developing osteoporosis by three times.

After menopause, talk to your doctor about taking estrogen. Estrogen-treated menopausal women have a much lower incidence of vertebral fractures. Postmenopausal women, especially, should have a regular program of weight-bearing exercise. Research now shows that such exercise not only maintains bone mass, it actually *increases* it, laying down additional minerals in the bones.

Treatment. Once you have osteoporosis, estrogen may not reverse the bone loss, but it will help to prevent further bone loss. Also, to prevent additional bone loss, you should take calcium supplements including calcium hydroxy apatite in the formula, recently shown to increase bone density, and you should eat a diet high in calcium. Sometimes supplements of vitamin D are also needed to ensure absorption of calcium by the body. (Check with your doctor for the proper amount, since vitamin D can accumulate in the body and result in toxic levels.) Lecithin may help the body use calcium and help maintain hormone balance.

In advanced osteoporosis a hormone called calcitonin is used to help prevent further bone loss and fractures. Orally administered bisphosphonates are also sometimes given. A drug called etidronate (Didronel), which in the past had been shown to be helpful in preventing further loss of calcium from bone, has now been shown to be able to actually *reverse* bone loss. In a two-year study in seven medical centers across the United States, women with osteoporosis who took the drug cut their risk of broken vertebrae in half. The drug, taken cyclically, several weeks on and several weeks off, has fewer side effects than does calcitonin.

Fluroide tablets, currently recommended almost routinely for osteoporosis, may not be given so routinely in the future. Researchers at the Mayo Clinic found that women who took fluoride had more fractures than women who did not. Meanwhile researchers at the University of Texas Southwestern Medical Center at Dallas find that slow-release sodium fluoride plus calcium citrate *will* increase bone strength. However, more research still needs to be done.

Losing excess weight is often beneficial since it decreases the burden on the bones and leads to more physical activity.

Osteomalacia

Researchers estimate that 20 percent of older persons in the United States with osteoporosis also have *softening* of the bone, called osteomalacia. It is primarily due to deficiency of vitamin D and calcium in the diet or to a problem in their absorption and metabolism in the body.

Anyone who does not get much sunlight risks developing osteomalacia unless they take vitamin D supplements, as do persons who have had part of their stomach removed, who have kidney, pancreas or liver disorders, or who take certain anticonvulsant drugs over long periods.

Bone pain may range from a dull ache to severe pain, usually beginning with pain in the lower back. When pressure is applied to affected bones, there is tenderness. The person may have difficulty climbing stairs or may have a waddling gait. The disease is often mistaken for osteoporosis or arthritis.

Treatment consists of a diet strong in milk, eggs, butter or margarine. Calcium and vitamin D supplements are also needed, with the calcium balanced in the proper ratio with other minerals, such as magnesium. In some cases, phosphorus is also needed.

Any major deformities may have to be corrected by traction or surgery, or both.

Rickets

Rickets is the same as osteomalacia—a faulty laying down of minerals because of a vitamin D deficiency—but it occurs in children instead of adults. The growing bone does not become properly calcified. Like osteomalacia, rickets can develop because of poor diet, because a child does not get the sunshine necessary for the absorption of vitamin D, or because of some problem with metabolism or digestion that interferes with the body's absorption and utilization of vitamin D. The abnormalities can occur in any bones, including the spine.

Infants with rickets are restless and sleep poorly, often developing a bald spot on the head from moving constantly in their sleep. Diagnosis is made by X ray, which shows the changes in the bones.

Treatment consists of daily vitamin D supplements that usually lead to improvement within days. After about one month, doses can be reduced to maintenance levels.

"Slipped Disc" and Other Spine Problems

First of all, there is no such thing as a "slipped disc." Discs don't slip. They may bulge or rupture, and thus cause pain, but they don't slip.

Discs are the gel-like pads made of cartilage, water, and

other substances that separate the vertebrae and—like the shock absorbers on your car—help to absorb the everyday shocks to your spine when you walk, run, sit, or do just about any other kind of activity. Trouble can start from a sudden injury, from long-term stress and strain, or from degenerative changes that occur over the years.

The Degenerated Disc

Discs lose much of their water content and become flatter as we grow older, the reason that most of us lose height in old age. Degeneration of the discs can occur in the vertebrae of the neck, the upper back, or lower back.

Back pain from disc degeneration typically begins with mild back pain. The patient recalls that after periods of prolonged physical activity or working in a position that causes stress to the spine, pain appears in the lower back. The pain lasts only a few days and then subsides. With the passage of time, the episodes may become more frequent and more intense. A trivial incident, even sneezing or coughing or stooping to pick up a handkerchief from the floor, may precipitate a severe attack.

(Note: In 1988 because of the much better imaging from magnetic resonance scanning, physicians began to see young people with low back pain who had dehydration, tears, or other deformities of degeneration of the spinal discs. Doctors named the newly recognized condition *juvenile discogenic disease*, or JDD. Strangely, it can occur in young people who are otherwise trim, fit, and physically active, who often are participants in sports. Drs. Charles Burton and Kenneth Heithoff, of Minneapolis, two of the early discoverers of the condition, say that JDD may turn out to be an early way to predict back problems likely to come in later life.)

The Bulging Disc

Some bulging is normal; just as a cushion bulges slightly

when you sit on it, your discs bulge when your spine exerts pressure on them. But other bulging is not normal, when the disc bulges and doesn't return to its resting shape but bulges out permanently and too far. It may protrude so far that it stretches the tiny nerves going to and from the ring around the disc (called the annulus). When these nerves are stretched, it causes pain in your back or your hip. (In some cases the pain can also form inflammation of the soft tissue in the area.)

Sometimes the disc bulges out so far that it pushes against one of the 31 major spinal nerves that go from each side of your spinal cord to the rest of your body. When the bulging disc pushed against one of these nerves, or pinches it in some way, you get radiating pain (called radiculopathy) in whatever part of your body that is supplied by that nerve. (This radiating pain can also be produced by an infection, a bony spur pushing against the nerve, or pressure from a tumor.) Typically there is a deep ache or sharp, stabbing pain that runs down the buttocks and hip to the thigh, with stiffness when bending forward. Any sudden jolt of the spine can cause searing pain.

Doctors measure the bulging in millimeters and talk about "a 1-mm bulge" or "2-mm bulge." The larger the bulge, the greater your symptoms.

Whether pain is produced also depends on how large or small the opening is where the nerve courses through the vertebrae to the rest of the body. If it is wide open, the nerve will be able to escape the bulging and there will be no pain. But if the opening is narrow (called spinal stenosis) and crowded by a spur or other problems, then the nerve cannot move out of the way.

Sometimes in addition to pain in the leg or arm, there may be other signs: loss of sense of touch in the area, lowered skin temperature of one area, weakness of a muscle such as that of the big toe, diminished knee-jerk or ankle-jerk reflexes, or pain produced or increased by coughing, sneezing, or bearing down.

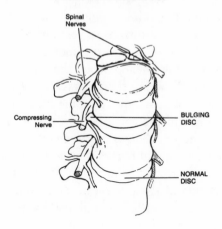

A NORMAL AND A BULGING DISC

The radiating pain is what many people—including some doctors—call sciatica. But this term, just like "slipped disc," is also out of date. The sciatic nerve is actually made up of several nerves that go to and along the muscles and skin of the legs and feet. We are going to teach you the pathways of each of the *separate* spinal nerves so that you, working with your doctor, can determine *exactly* where the problem is coming from in your spine. Then you will know you have a problem in your spine at the level of, say, the fourth lumbar nerve, instead of the vague term "sciatica."

The Ruptured Disc

There is another thing that can happen: the bulge can grow larger and larger and become weak and the ring around the disc—the annulus—can rupture, allowing the gel-like nucleus of the disc to partly stick out. The nucleus sticking out of the ruptured disc can press against the spinal nerves and cause even worse pain than the simple bulging disc.

Free Fragments

Sometimes the contents of the disc can come out, floating loose and free in the spinal cavity. When this happens, pressure against a spinal nerve sometimes is released and pain decreases, but sometimes the free fragment can float to other areas in the spinal canal and cause even more complications.

Treatment When You Have an Acute Disc Attack

Rest in bed. Only if you are lying down is the disc free of significant stress. When you are lying down, your discs expand, pressure is removed, and nutrients diffuse into the area, all of which helps to ease pain and aid healing. Sitting does not provide the same relief.

Your physician may give you a drug to reduce inflammation and reduce the pressure enough to eradicate pain, or a muscle relaxant if there is muscle spasm, or a pain-reliever. Remember if you take any of these drugs, you still need bedrest.

Manipulation is sometimes helpful. If you have it, keep your muscles and joints moving afterward, don't hold them in one position; and take a warm bath with water shoulder-high to keep muscles relaxed.

After an attack no heavy work or exercise should be done without the approval of your doctor.

Spondylolysis

In this condition there is a breakdown of the bony structure of one of the vertebra, sometimes from an inborn anatomical weakness or sometimes caused by injury or stress, such as in soldiers who carry heavy backpacks or persons performing exercises they are not accustomed to.

Back-strengthening exercises are helpful. Most people with the condition can engage in mild sports and activities, but should avoid vigorous activities, such as football, that could cause injury. Persons with spondylolysis should have annual X rays to check on the condition.

Some people have the condition and never develop symptoms. In others, it can lead to spondylolisthesis.

Spondylolisthesis

This condition occurs when one vertebra slides forward and overhangs the vertebra below it. It often first occurs during the rapid growth period of childhood, usually between ages 5 and 17, but the person may have no back complaint until perhaps age 35, when a sudden twisting or lifting brings on pain. Some people, even with a significant degree of slipping, will have no discomfort whatsoever and will be astonished if the slippage of the vertebra is found on a routine X ray.

If symptoms do occur, they are usually aggravated by strenuous activity and will be relieved by rest.

One diagnostic clue is when the person often has tightness of the hamstring muscles in the legs, with a typical posture of bending slightly forward with flexed hips and knees. He or she may have difficulty raising a leg without bending the knee. There may be a strange stiff-legged way of walking.

For an acute attack, bedrest and aspirin or other anti-inflammatory medicine are often helpful. A corset can be used to support the weakened spinal area when needed. A medically supervised program of exercises like the ones in this book may help to prevent further damage. If exercise is not successful, surgery may be necessary. The person who begins to have symptoms should do no heavy lifting or prolonged or repetitive bending.

Facet Syndrome

A vertebral facet is the surface of one of the bony knobs that sticks out on a vertebra where it meets a knob on another vertebra. They make a sort of arch to protect your nerves where they branch off the spinal cord to go to the rest of the body. If the vertebrae get out of line—because of degenerated discs, for example—then one vertebra can slide forward or back on the other, causing abnormal stress on the joint and irritation. If there is enough irritation, tiny spinal muscles can go into spasm or bony spurs can be formed, both of which can cause pain, or the reduced size of the opening can crowd the nerve, causing pain.

There may be tenderness over one or more of the joints, referred pain over the buttock or thigh, or worsening of pain when sitting in one position a long time, but these symptoms may occur with other back problems too, so diagnosis is often difficult.

Diagnosis is usually made by injecting local anesthetic into the joint of the vertebra. Relief of pain confirms the diagnosis.

Usual treatment is a NSAID medication and rest. If this does not work, the same injection that confirms the diagnosis often will work as effective treatment. Sometimes surgery is necessary.

CHAPTER FOURTEEN

When Surgery Is Necessary

It is estimated that approximately 450,000 back surgeries are performed each year, costing patients, their families, and their employers billions of dollars in surgical and disability expenses.

It's a frightening time when the doctor tells you that you need to have back surgery. You are so tired of the pain you could cry, but you are so afraid of surgery that you don't want to say yes to it.

It's a difficult decision. However, the good news is that there are many new techniques in surgery that make back surgery easier, safer, and more effective, especially the new, exciting ones that are giving such good results at the Institute.

When It Comes to Surgery, You May Want Another Opinion

Let's say a surgeon has made a recommendation to you for surgery. If you have not already been in touch with your family doctor about this problem, you should do so for his or her opinion. Does your own physician agree that surgery is indicated? Who do they think is best suited for performing the operation? Consider also getting an independent opinion from another qualified surgeon.

Have your family doctor *and* your surgeon explain to you the alternatives to surgery, the potential benefits, and possible complications of the various alternatives.

Discuss in detail how much relief of pain your doctor expects the surgery to give you. Sometimes surgery will give complete relief; in other cases, patients can only expect partial relief, or relief of leg pain not back pain.

On the other hand, don't push a doctor into performing surgery if he or she does not think it is needed.

When Should Surgery Be Done?

If you have unbearably severe pain and there are symptoms of nerve damage, such as bladder or bowel disturbances, or paralysis of any muscles, this is called cauda equina syndrome and calls for emergency surgery—*immediately*, within hours.

Otherwise, surgery should be done only after a thorough exercise program and other more conservative measures as outlined in this book have been tried. Only after these don't work should surgery be done.

Before You Have Surgery

Even after you have decided to go ahead with surgery, unless it is an emergency, we strongly recommend that you use whatever time you have before your surgery is performed to continue diligently to follow an exercise program as prescribed by your doctor. If at the time of your scheduled operation you still have severe pain, and if your doctor still strongly recommends surgery, then do not put surgery off any longer, because further delay is of no benefit. The exercises done before surgery can then help the back to return faster to normal function and strength after surgery.

Even after surgery it is still important to do exercises (check with your surgeon for the right ones for you) to help build back the strength of your back. In fact, patients who have surgery usually will have occasional back trouble if they do not follow up with a sustained exercise program like the one in this book. At GCOC we schedule all our postsurgery patients for six weeks of physical therapy and individualized exercise (including pool exercises).

Note: Because we can't know every reader's individual medical situation, be sure to get your doctor's approval for the exercises and work your exercises with his or her guidance.

What to Do Before and After Surgery to Reduce Complications and to Recover Faster

- If you are a smoker, stop smoking before surgery—the earlier the better.
- If you drink alcohol, stop drinking for several weeks before going in for surgery.
- Do not take aspirin or any aspirin products for several weeks beforehand.
- If you come down with a cold or other respiratory infection, postpone the surgery.
- If there is time, have loose or infected teeth treated.
- Get plenty of rest and nourishing foods for the weeks preceding an operation.
- Check with your doctor on the back exercises he or she especially wants you to do, or not do, before the surgery.
- Discuss with your doctor taking supplements of zinc, vitamins A and C, and bioflavanoids for several weeks before

surgery and during the recovery period, all of which have been shown to speed healing.

- Tell your doctor about any chronic disease or allergies that you have, and about any medicine you take. If you have any blood problems, such as anemia, or any allergies to medications, tell both the surgeon and the anesthesiologist.
- Talk to your doctor about how soon you can move around and exercise. Even in bed you can do contractions of your feet and leg muscles. Sit up and walk as soon as your doctor says you can. This will not only help you heal faster, it will also help prevent blood clots from forming in your leg veins. If you have had general anesthesia, yawn a lot afterward to help inflate the lungs and prevent the pulmonary complications that sometimes occur after general anesthesia.

Kinds of Surgery

Discectomy (Partial Removal of a Disc)

This is the most common kind of back surgery.

If a disc is degenerated or ruptured or pressing on a nerve, it can cause excruciating pain. Removing part of the disc can relieve the pressure and the cause of the pain.

Nuclectomy

This refers to the delicate removal of part of the *nucleus* of the disc. The outer covering (*annulus fibrosis*) of the disc is penetrated, and with a small forceps some of the inside gel-like material (the nucleus) is removed. This allows for the decompression of the area, much as removal of part of the disc would.

Laminectomy

In a laminectomy the surgeon removes a part of the vertebra, the bony section that makes up the arch. This is usually done to remove a disc or to remove loose fragments that have ruptured from the disc. It is also used when the patient has *spinal stenosis*, an unusual narrowing of the space (the tunnel for the spinal cord) making up the spinal canal. Some people are born with a narrow spinal canal; others have a buildup of bone spurs or other factors that narrow the spinal canal. (These spurs can be produced by arthritis, injury, obesity, old operations, degenerative changes or by abnormal pressures on the vertebra forcing a bit of the bone to hang over and stick out into the spinal canal.) The surgeon removes whatever is blocking the canal, giving more room for the nerve roots.

Foramenostomy

This is a procedure for removing a spur, scar tissue, or adhesions from old operations that could be narrowing the foramen (the opening through which nerve roots pass).

Facet Denervation

Facets are the little flat surfaces of the vertebrae where the vertebrae join each other and form the foramen for the nerve roots to come in and go out of the spinal cord. As discs settle, the pressure on the facet joints can wear down cartilage and cause arthritic changes. Facet denervation is a technique that destroys the tiny branches of the nerves going to the facets. The technique is also called *facet rhizotomy*.

It may be that many patients diagnosed as having "slipped disc" are wrongly diagnosed—what they really have is disturbances in the facet joints and the nerve branches there.

The term *facet syndrome* can also refer to the facets catching on each other because of bony outgrowths. The destruction of the tiny nerves going to the facets is effective to correct the problem in many back patients.

Spinal Fusion

If a joint is unstable and slips, causing pinching of a nerve root, spinal fusion can be done as a last resort. In fusion, two or three joints are fused together by joining two vertebrae with a bone graft. Bone chips are usually taken from another part of the body (usually the hip or pelvic bone) and grafted or joined to the weak or damaged vertebrae to form a nonflexible section of the spine. Freeze-dried donor bone and synthetic materials are also used. Sometimes metal plates, wires, or screws are used for reinforcement. The rest of the back remains flexible and you are able to bend and move normally. The success rate of fusion of the vertebra with the implanted bone can sometimes be increased by stimulating the area with an electromagnetic field. Some fusions involve the insertion of a stainless steel rod along the affected area of the spine to help hold the spine rigid while the bone graft heals. The technique is useful when there is weakness of a vertebrae or two, but fusing one level does not protect other levels of the spine. In fact, there often is weakening of the joints above and below the level where the fusion was done. Only when there is spinal instability and when motion aggravates pain is fusion likely to help a patient. The scientific name for fusion is *arthrodesis*. Usually, for several months after fusion, the patient is not allowed to ride in a car or sit for long periods.

(You may also come across the term *ankylosis*. This refers to the fusion of two joints that occurs naturally, not by surgery.)

Chemonucleolysis—The Enzyme Treatment

Chymopapain, an enzyme derived from the papaya plant, is used by some surgeons to relieve the symptoms caused by a bulging disc. The medical name for the technique is chemonucleolysis. It involves injection of the enzyme, via a long needle, into the affected disc, with careful placement using an X-ray monitor. The enzyme breaks down the gel-like material within the disc, which then is absorbed into the body. The disc, now skinnier, slips back into place between the vertebrae, eliminating the pressure on the nerves that was causing pain. The average hospital stay is about three days.

Chemonucleolysis gets mixed reviews. The technique was used in the United States from 1969 to 1975. About three out of four patients were helped, but there were many side effects, including two deaths, and its use in the United States was halted. But the technique was in great demand by the public, and since then many patients have traveled to Canada and other countries to have it done. After several years a study was done of a new version of the technique which showed a better record, and the FDA released the enzyme for general use in the United States. By the end of 1985 some 90,000 patients had been injected. But there were still dangerous complications— serious allergic reactions, sometimes paralysis or other neurological complications, even deaths. Especially dangerous was when some patients had a general allergic reaction (*anaphylaxis*). The treatment continued to be used in Europe, but in the United States it dropped to only 5 percent of its former use. Strangely enough in Europe there were fewer allergic reactions. One theory for this is the frequent use of papain as a meat tenderizer in American cooking, so that more people became allergic to it.

Now several things have happened to bring chemonucleolysis back into wider use. The technique was improved so that injections will not inadvertently go into other areas of the spine. The problem of allergic reactions was greatly helped by excluding patients with an allergic history, by testing patients for sensitivity to the enzyme before surgery, and by reducing the dosage of enzyme.

The International Intradiscal Therapy Society, a professional group of some 200 surgeons who use the technique, says that chemonucleolysis has been about 80 percent effective in the more than 240,000 patients worldwide who have now received it since the 1960s. There have been no deaths since 1987. One research group in Japan is now investigating the use of disc injections with corticosteroids.

The chemonucleolysis technique is used *only* for treating a bulging disc. It will not work for back pain due to arthritis, pulled muscles, or other causes or even for discs from which there has already been a rupture of material. You should not have the enzyme treatment if you are allergic to meat tenderizer, papaya, or beer because you may be allergic to the enzyme. It should not be used in pregnant women.

If you do choose this option, you should find a surgeon who has a great deal of experience with it, ask that the lowest possible dose be used, and make sure you are tested for possible allergy to the enzyme before surgery. Have the surgery under local anesthesia, so that if there are any signs of the beginnings of an allergic reaction such as nausea, itching, or dizziness, you can immediately tell the surgeon. Because of the potential of having developed sensitivity, do not ever have the procedure repeated a second time.

Microsurgery

In the past to operate on the back, a large incision had to be made, and much tissue had to be cut and bone removed to reach the places that needed repair. Microsurgery has helped solve much of that, and can be used to remove a disc (microdiscectomy). The surgery is performed through an incision about half an inch to an inch long, with procedures being viewed through an operating microscope. This was a step forward, with less trauma to patients, fewer complications, and shorter hospital stays than the standard large open-wound laminectomy.

The Newest Surgery—Arthroscopy and Other Percutaneous Surgery for the Back

"I'm tired of the pain... I've lived with it six years... I can't take it any more," says one New Jersey housewife.

199

From a nurse: "I used to lift patients from wheelchair to bed, and my back finally gave out. I've had two open surgeries on my back, including fusion, but I still hurt."

From an accountant: "I was in a serious car accident. My doctor told me I would have to get used to the idea that I would be crippled and in pain for the rest of my life."

A letter carrier who slipped on an icy sidewalk says he has been unable to carry mailbags for two months. His wife, hit by a truck and left on the road, has been in a wheelchair and in excruciating pain for three months.

A helicopter pilot, who was in a helicopter crash in 1970, says he has had three operations and every time he moves "It feels like something is stabbing me." When he turns his neck, a grinding noise is heard. He takes pain medicine every day and wakes up with pain every night. His doctor told him he had a hostile attitude and would have to live with the pain.

These are all patients telling their stories in the waiting room of the GCOC Institute. And they all subsequently had arthroscopic or other percutaneous surgery and were quickly and safely relieved of their pain.

These new techniques have brought us to a new era in back surgery. Today, with the new simpler and safer arthroscopic techniques, we can do surgery earlier, and so alleviate problems *before* they become disabling. These procedures can be done on an outpatient basis with no anesthesia except for numbing of the skin and just minimal discomfort. In about 30 minutes we can have people back to an almost normal condition with no transfusions, no hospital stays, no medications.

Percutaneous surgery was the first development of these wonderful new techniques. *Percutaneous* refers to surgical procedures done through a tiny hole placed in the skin (about ⅛ inch). The idea of inserting instruments through a hole to reach in to the discs of the spine was in the minds of surgeons about 20 years ago, but it took the development of CAT scanning and magnetic resonance imaging so that surgeons could properly determine the location of problems in the spine and see how to approach them to make the idea a reality.

Some of the first work was done by Dr. Sadahisa Hijikata, of Keio University School of Medicine in Tokyo. Research in the United States on the technique was begun in the mid-1980s by Dr. Gary Onik and others of the Allegheny General Hospital in Pittsburgh, by the GCOC Institute, and by a medical team at the University of California, San Francisco.

Percutaneous Automated Discectomy (PAD)

The first application of the technique was percutaneous automated discectomy (PAD), removing parts of a bulging disc that was pressing against a spinal nerve, or removing some of the disc interior, allowing the disc to retreat back into its proper location between the vertebra, so that it would no longer push against a nerve root and cause pain.

Here is how percutaneous discectomy (sometimes called *nuclectomy*) is done: After the skin is anesthetized with novocaine so that it is numb, a specially designed stainless steel instrument— hollow like a soda straw—is used to make a hole in the skin and is slowly and carefully directed by the surgeon to the damaged disc while he watches the exact location of the instrument on an X-ray machine. The X-ray camera is on a long, C-shaped arm that can move above, below, or around the operating table during surgery to get views of the spine area from any angle. When the instrument is snug against the covering of the disc, a slightly larger hollow instrument—this time with a tiny knife inside—is inserted. A small cut is made in the membrane of the disc, and small pieces of disc material are suctioned from the interior into the instrument. The supporting structure of the disc is not affected. During the entire procedure, the patient is awake and alert, sometimes watching the procedure on the TV monitor, so that he or she can inform the surgeon of decrease or increase of pain, or any pain or tingling in the legs that might be due to the probe getting too close to the spinal cord or to a spinal nerve. Upon completion, the instrument is removed and only a Band-Aid is needed over the instrument hole.

Helen was a 26-year-old dental assistant who could hardly walk and could not sleep because of severe pain in her back and down her legs. She was given conservative treatment of bedrest, anti-inflammatory drugs, and an exercise program. She was evaluated with X rays, magnetic resonance imaging (MRI), and other tests to locate the offending areas and was scheduled for surgery. An hour and a half after percutaneous discectomy surgery, she smilingly thanked the staff and showed them how well she could walk. She is back at work now.

Another woman, brought in by her family, had not walked in six months, but hours after surgery she walked using a walker, and then in a few days without it. The patient's family, in the waiting room, was able to watch the operation on closed-circuit television. (All surgeries are recorded for evaluation and case studies, so patients can see their own surgery after it is over.)

The percutaneous discectomy procedure is now being used by a number of surgeons in Europe and the United States. At GCOC we have now performed the percutaneous discectomy procedure for more than three years on over 400 patients, from ages 24 to 76. If we get to the disc early enough—when it is only bulging 2 to 3 mm into the vertebral space and it is in middle and lower back—we obtain good results in 100 percent of patients. When the patient comes in for surgery after the condition has progressed—when the disc has bulged to 3 to 4 mm and the pain going down the legs has become excruciating— there are good results in about 80–90 percent. "Good results" means the patient is totally free of pain and has returned to normal function. The procedure does not work well when the disc has protruded more than 4 mm, especially in the area between the last lumbar and the first sacral vertebra.

The percutaneous discectomy technique is designed for patients who have not responded to conventional treatment, who have radiating leg pain, and whose CAT scan or MRI and other tests have shown that there is a bulging spinal disc in the low back area. It does not work in cases that are so advanced that the disc has ruptured and there are free fragments of disc tissue floating in the spinal canal—a reason for not putting off surgery. If you postpone surgery when there is severe radiating pain and a bulging disc has been shown to be the cause, the disc may rupture, and this simple technique can no longer be used.

Percutaneous Foramenostomy

Percutaneous foramenostomy has just recently been added to what can be done through the skin. The widening of the opening for nerve roots can be done in patients who have pain due to spinal stenosis (narrowing of the spinal foramen opening between the vertebrae) or who have spurs or entrapment of nerves in areas of adhesions or scars from previous surgeries.

This technique was also developed at GCOC, and we had to design special instruments to do the procedure that could slip around spinal nerves and between the bones of the spine and reach the inner areas where the narrowing pain-causing problems were. We now have developed a variety of miniaturized operating tools, such as a tiny impactor, miniature knives and scissors, and a grasper for the removal of loose bodies and fragments of tissue. They are designed to all telescope into one unit so only one entry point is needed and the surgeon can maneuver and perform the procedure with minimal discomfort to the patient.

In this operation, a probe is used to penetrate to the desired area, any excess disc material is removed to reduce pressure in the area, and then any spurs or other things that are narrowing the space and crowding the nerve are loosened with a tiny impactor and removed.

In these cases—about 100 have been done so far on patients ages 17 to 92—the patient experiences almost complete relief of pain as soon as any inflammation goes away. In these first cases, we have obtained good results of pain relief in 85 percent. There were no postoperative complications. The results in more recent patients continues to be excellent.

Arthroscopy of the Back

Arthroscopy was the next technique developed to go along with the percutaneous approach. In arthroscopy (arthros'ko-pee), a tiny fiber optic lens and lighting system is inserted through the opening in the skin and into the *inside* of the joint where it illuminates and magnifies the structures inside the joint so that the doctor can look at a television monitor and see the view that the lens sees in the vertebral joint, to see the location of what is causing pain, and to see exactly what is happening as he works with the internal surgical procedure. The tiny instrument is only about ¼ inch in diameter.

With a view of the arthroscopic camera right in the joint on one monitor screen and the X-ray view on the other monitor, it makes it much easier to see what is happening and to be in control of the most delicate maneuvers.

One typical patient, a 29-year-old woman who had been in a serious car accident, had severe back pain and pain in both legs that started within hours of the accident. She had been on constant painkillers and muscle relaxants, but the pain continued, and she had not been able to work for three months by the time she was referred to GCOC. Her MRI study showed that she had a severely bulging disc. She was operated on and returned to work in three weeks and has been free of pain ever since.

A 23-year-old carpenter also was referred after a car accident. He could walk no more than one city block before excruciating pain hit him. The pain was in his lower back area and radiated to his right side, going down his thigh, to his calf and the top of this foot. (The lumbar area is most frequently involved in back pain because it carries most of the body's stresses.) His MRI study also showed a bulging disc. As the material from the bulging disc was removed under arthroscopy, he said that the constant pain he had been experiencing—right as we were operating—suddenly disappeared. Two hours after surgery he went home, and two weeks later he went back to work, with the advice to not lift heavy loads or strain his back, but otherwise to work normally. He is still pain free.

At the GCOC Institute we now do almost all our operations on the back using the arthroscope and have recently given a report to a surgical meeting on the first 1,000 patients.

The development of arthroscopy for the back is parallel to the revolution in knee surgery 10 or 15 years ago. Before that, if someone had an injured knee that required surgery, it meant that the person would have general anesthesia, need a large incision, stay in the hospital a week or more, walk with crutches for perhaps two months, and for much of this time be in horrendous pain. People were afraid to have that surgery— with reason—and often those with bad knees preferred to suffer their pain and the certainty of later arthritis rather than have the surgery. Those seem like dinosaur days. Now we can use an arthroscope and do knee surgery in half an hour, and the patient can be walking and in no pain the next day.

Now the same revolution has just begun in back surgery.

We're also, in conjunction with arthroscopy, beginning to use laser surgery, a wonderfully delicate and easy-to-use technique that has been used for eye surgery in the last few years, and just now is being developed for back surgery.

The big advantage of these techniques is that there is no long recovery period—the patient returns to full activity and his or her job in an amazingly short time. In addition, there are very few risks to the patient. There is no large incision, no muscle dissection, no manipulation of nerves, no bone removal as in standard open back surgery, and almost no bleeding and no formation of scar tissue that might cause future problems. Because there is almost no injury to the tissue, there is very little pain, and healing is fast. The tiny freckle-sized puncture wound, as opposed to an open incision, means there is less risk of infection and other complications. The procedure is also cheaper, since it can be performed in 30–40 minutes on an outpatient basis, so that hospitalization is not needed. Nor is general anesthesia needed (but an anesthesiologist is present to control and direct the patient during the procedure, and sometimes a tranquilizer is given).

The patient often feels relief from pain immediately following the procedure, sometimes even on the operating table. No postsurgical medication is needed. In the recovery room, where they stay for two to three hours, patients are usually treated with an ice pack on the area and electrical stimulation from a transcutaneous electrical nerve stimulation (TENS) unit. Usually no postoperative medication is needed. Walking is permitted the same day. Patients are checked at home that evening by a nurse, return the next day for an evaluation, and are evaluated again at one week; they follow a physical therapy program for three to six weeks, and have other evaluations and treatments as indicated.

Most patients are able to return to active daily living, with some restrictions, within days. After one month, most patients are able to return to work with minimum restrictions. At the end of three months, most are released from further checkups or treatments, with no restrictions in activity or job. The procedure is better, less risky, less traumatic, and less costly than open spine surgery.

(With a new variation of the procedure developed at GCOC for neck problems, approximately 80 percent of 200 neck patients operated on thus far also have experienced pain relief.)

How You Can Help Your Surgeon Find Where Your Pain Is Coming From

Remember when we said that we think the term "sciatica" should be abolished? The reason is that we have the knowledge now to tell in most patients exactly where a bulging disc, a spur, or other abnormality is causing the pain. The key is using a chart of the pathways of the nerves coming from the spinal cord. Each goes to a specific area, so that when you determine in exactly what area your pain, numbness, or weakness is felt, you and your surgeon will know where the pain is coming from. When your pain patterns are compared with the evidence of the X ray and the MRI and other diagnostic tests, and they all match in saying what is causing the problem, then the surgeon knows exactly where to go into the spine to remove the disc bulge or spur to correct the problem.

Then instead of saying "I have lumbago or sciatica," you can talk about having "an L4 nerve problem" (the fourth lumbar nerve) or "nerve involvement of L5" (the fifth lumbar nerve) or "S1" (the first sacral nerve). The patients at GCOC become quite knowledgeable about their condition and can pinpoint exact patterns for the doctor. They understand what their problem is, what is going to be done for it, and whether the procedure has worked.

Learning about your pain patterns can be one of the most important things you do toward understanding your particular back pain. It is so simple, and it can be a major key to feeling that you are in control of your situation. We use it with every single back patient who comes to the Institute.

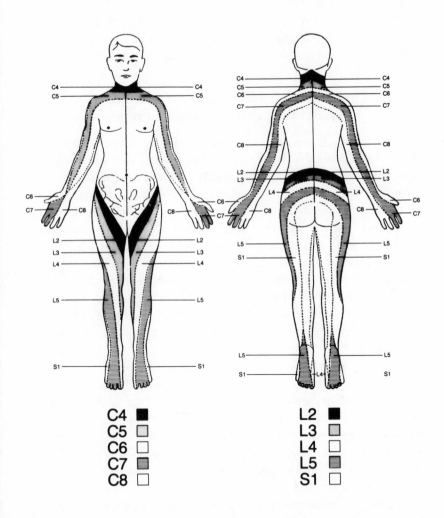

NERVE PATHWAYS

Pain Patterns

Look at the chart on page 208. Each different area refers to the pathway of a specific nerve.

Do you have pain down the inside of the arm, but not the hand? It probably is due to a problem in the spine at C5. Do you have pain down the side of the arm and to the thumb? The problem is probably at C6. Does the pain go to the fingers? It probably is a problem at C7 or C8.

Or maybe you have pain in the leg. Is it on the back in the area of the calf muscle and to the little toe? It's probably from a problem at S1. Or does it go across the back and around to your upper thigh? It's probably from a problem at L2. Or if it follows down from the outside of your thigh to the inside, it could be L3 or L4. But if it goes over your knee and down to your big toe, it's probably from a problem at L4. Or does it go from your lower back down your shin and to the middle toes? It's probably a problem at L5.

The spinal nerve comes out of the space just above it. So if the X ray shows a bulging disc in the space between L3 and L4, you probably will be showing the pattern of the L4 nerve.

Sometimes it's very clear-cut. Other times more than one disc is involved so there will be an overlap in patterns, and not be so simple to interpret. But with these clues, you can almost always make a guess as to the location level of what is causing the trouble.

If there is more than one problem area, the surgeon deals only with one level at one operating time, because often solving the problem at one level will give enough space for the vertebrae to spread out a little and relieve the pressure that is causing pain from other pinched nerves. (Remember the helicopter pilot with the terrible neck? He had to go in twice for surgery to correct two different problems at two different levels. The first operation relieved some, but not all, of the pain. The second operation eliminated the rest.)

Confimatory Tests

As a second set of clues, the surgeon will also do some confirmatory tests such as checking knee reflexes and strength of the grip of your hand or how well you can resist the pushing up or down of your foot. These are to test for weakness of muscles or disappearance of nerve reflexes in specific areas, again being a clue to confirm the level in the spine causing the problem. When all these clues come together, the surgeon knows exactly where to go in and what to do.

You can use some of these tests on yourself if you have pain radiating down to your hip or legs. The most common nerve involvements are L4, L5, and S1, because that is where most of the motion of the spine occurs and that is where there is the most potential for breakdown.

The Knee-Jerk Test for L4 To test the knee jerk (patellar tendon reflex), sit on a table or chair with legs dangling or with one leg crossed over the other knee. Have someone use a rubber hammer or the edge of his hand to quickly tap the tendon just under your kneecap at the knee joint. Your leg should jump up involuntarily. Repeat the procedure on the other leg, and compare the two. If the knee-jerk reflex is missing on the same leg where you have radiating pain coming over the knee and down to the big toe, you very likely have L4 nerve involvement.

Toe Flexion Test for L5 When the fifth lumbar nerve root is pinched at the spine, it affects the muscles that extend your ankle and raise your toes. You can test this by trying to resist when someone pushes down on your toes while holding your ankle. If you cannot resist, and you have pain going from the hip down the leg to the middle three toes, it is very likely involvement of the fifth nerve.

Ankle-Jerk Test for S1 To test for the ankle jerk (Achilles tendon reflex), sit on the edge of a table with legs dangling. Have someone hold your foot up a little, then using a rubber hammer or a hand, have him sharply tap the tendon running down the back of your ankle. Your foot should jump up involuntarily. Test the ankle of the other leg, and compare.

Another test for S1 is to try to walk on your toes. If you are

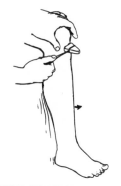

KNEE JERK TEST

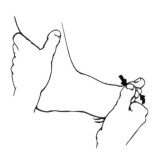

TOE FLEXION TEST

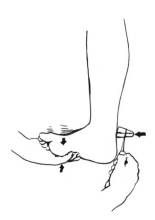

ANKLE JERK TEST

unable to do so, it indicates weakness of the calf muscle, another sign of S1 involvement. Or try to stand on one leg and rise up on your toes five times in succession. Inability to do this also indicates calf muscle weakness. If these tests show weakness and you have pain coming from the hip down the back of the legs and to the little toe, there probably is involvement of the first sacral nerve, the one coming up through the space at L5/S1.

A typical case was a 76-year-old woman who had a gradual onset of discomfort and pain in the back, which became progressively worse, until it extended down the back of her thigh and calf, to her heel and little toe. (Aha! S1!) The pain was constant and kept her awake at night. An X ray and an MRI study showed that she had several bulging discs, the worst one being between L5 and S1. (Aha again!) It was confirmed by weakness in her calf and loss of her ankle-jerk reflex. Neither bedrest nor traction eased her pain, so she was scheduled for arthroscopic discectomy, and within two hours was able to walk and went home. At three- and six-week checkups, she was found to be free of discomfort and pain and has remained free of all symptoms.

The system works wonderfully, and accurately. If you have back pain with radiating pain in the arms and legs, study the charts to see what pattern your pain follows, and if you wish, do some of the confirmatory muscle and reflex tests. Then discuss the pattern and the severity of the pain (use a scale of 1 to 10) with your doctor. This also gives you an excellent way to measure your improvement after surgery.

The Future for Back Surgery

People have been afraid of back surgery because of the horrendous disasters that we all have heard about. Sometimes the result of surgery was worse than the original problems. And every one out five operations failed to get results.

But now we are dealing with a new world. Key surgeons in centers in several countries throughout the world are starting to use the new percutaneous techniques such as arthroscopy for the back.

We predict that ten years from now, they will be commonplace, making old surgery techniques for the back seem barbaric. Just as with knee surgery, it will be common for people to have back surgery and go back to their jobs within a few days. The terrible disasters, and the fears, are going to disappear.

The new techniques can help huge numbers of people get back to normal, active lives—pain-free—to start enjoying their lives again.

Never again will patients have to settle for being told "You'll have to learn to live with the pain."

The important thing, now that you know how many things can be done to help your back, is that you don't sit back and be helpless. You are the most important member of the medical team in the care of your back. And with the new advances in treatment, giving you a new chance with your back, you should do everything possible to make that second chance pay off so that you can have a future free of pain forever.

Emergency!
First Aid for the Injured Back

At the Scene of an Accident

Here are the proper procedures to follow if you find yourself at the scene of an accident where a person may have a spine injury.

- Send someone to summon a physician or an ambulance.
- Check to see if the victim is breathing. If not, provide mouth-to-mouth resuscitation.
- If there is extensive bleeding, apply clean cloths gently to stop bleeding.
- Cover the injured person to keep him or her warm and to help counteract shock.

Don't do anything else. Unless there is danger of fire or explosion, do not move the victim. Leave him or her at the site. Do not put a pillow under the victim's head. Do not bend or twist the victim in any way. Do not try to pull him or her out of a wrecked car or lift or move the person in any way unless danger of fire, explosion, or other imminent life-threatening condition exists.

Do not rush the victim to the hospital. Wait for an ambulance or paramedics to come to the victim.

If it is necessary to move the victim because of fire or other immediate danger or because no help is on the way, do it with great care to avoid any possibility of damage to the spinal cord. *Do not let the victim's head bend forward or tilt in any way.* Devise a rigid emergency stretcher such as a door or wide wooden plank. Put it alongside the victim, and have one person kneel and grasp the victim's head firmly between hands while others grasp the victim's clothing at hips and shoulder and slide the victim carefully onto the stretcher, moving the entire body and head as a unit with no bending. Put rolled towels or sweaters or other padding on the sides of the head to prevent rolling. Tie the person to the stretcher in several places. If an ambulance is not available and the victim must be transported, use a truck or station wagon with a flat floor (pad it if possible). The emphasis must be to keep the victim's body (spine) rigid and immobile. Drive *very slowly* since bumps or jolts can cause injury.

Test: To test for damage to the neck, if the victim is alert, tell the victim to not lift his or her head, but to tentatively tense their muscles as though trying to lift it. If pain is experienced there probably is serious damage to the neck.

In the Emergency Room

Whether the back injury patient is paralyzed for life or can be rehabilitated is determined not only by how he is treated at the scene of the accident, but also by how he is treated in the emergency room at the hospital. It is important that mistakes not be made during the period of emergency room medical care.

The primary rule in the early care of the patient with back injury is to avoid movement of the back, neck, and head. To be sure this rule isn't broken, try to accompany the patient to the hospital emergency or receiving room. Examination should be done while the patient is still on the stretcher, with the clothing being cut off to avoid the movement of undressing. Only after the patient is examined and immobilized should the patient be transferred from the stretcher.

If You Have Been in an Accident

Often people involved in car accidents don't go to the emergency room. That is a mistake. You should go to an emergency room of a hospital to have X rays of any areas that hurt. You may have hidden injuries, such as a hidden fracture, that an X ray will uncover. Or damage may show up later, and it is prudent to have on record for insurance purposes the fact that you had an accident and went to get care. Sometimes you may have had what seemed like a small jolt, but the next day be racked with pain all over.

Even if the emergency room examination shows no apparent damage, you should watch for delayed evidence of injury that could appear later that day, or even several days later.

Medical help should be obtained immediately if any of the following signs occur in someone who has had a head or back injury:

- Inability to move fingers, toes, or other parts of the body
- Tingling or numb feeling in any part of the body
- Blood or other fluid coming from mouth, ears, or nose
- Nausea or vomiting
- Disturbance in vision, such as double vision, blurring, or difficulty in focusing the eyes

- Unequal size of pupils of eyes or pupils that are very dilated or contracted to pinpoints
- Headache
- Unusual sleepiness or drowsiness with difficulty in rousing the person
- Convulsions or blanking-out episodes
- Difficulty in breathing
- Speech difficulties
- Strange behavior or changes in personality or mental ability

Sometimes a small hidden fracture can be missed in the emergency room; the doctor finds one spinal fracture and looks no further. However, where there's one spinal fracture, there often may be another. All patients with spinal cord injuries should get X rays of the entire spine right away. Additional hidden fractures might not generate symptoms at first, but later could turn out to be something very serious.

Hidden fractures can also sometimes occur even in a minor accident. Without your realizing it, a small part of one vertebra can break, especially if your bones are weakened by disease such as bone infection or osteoporosis. Fractures can occur even from such things as strenuous sports or falling and landing hard on your feet. Many such fractures go unrecognized when they happen and are only found later when the patient goes to the doctor with a complaint of persistent pain, or is not able to stand straight.

If you have suffered a back or spine injury as a result of an accident, and that accident was the fault of another party, you will most likely be contacted by an insurance adjuster or attorney representing that responsible party. In discussing payments to pay you for your injury and expenses, they may propose a final settlement and full release. In making your decision, remember that problems or complications sometimes develop days or weeks later where the neck and back are involved, so you may want to delay finalizing any settlement or release until you have discussed all possible problems with your physician.

Note: Check your present insurance policy. Often the personal injury allowance is only for $10,000; for a few dollars more, you can increase that to $200,000 coverage.

If You Are Hurt at Work

Once any emergency treatment is completed, if you were hurt at work, call your supervisor or your company's medical department to report the accident and to confirm that they know what has happened to you and that proper procedures have been begun by them for having someone handle your job and for processing the appropriate medical insurance forms.

In most cases payments are made for lost wages and medical bills without any problem within a few weeks, but sometimes the Worker's Compensation system is extremely slow. Patients are sent from doctor to doctor to doctor, in a maze of red tape, when they need treatment promptly.

If there is some dispute in your case, discuss the situation with your boss and the insurance company and also have your physician talk with them to make sure they completely understand all the facts in the case.

We Need a New System

It may be time for a new system of Worker's Compensation. We need to get patients sooner into the hands of a physician who can help them.

One way to do that would be if compensation time were limited. For a particular injury, you would be given a specified time for medical treatment, after which payment would stop and the patient would have to pay out of pocket for further treatments. As it stands now, we keep paying no matter how long the patient is in treatment and stays out of work. It motivates the patient in the wrong direction, and sometimes the patient goes for years without working.

There needs to be a classification of various injuries and the length of time that payments will be made for them, much as there is now for regular insurance payments for hospitalization so that physician and patient will put forth the maximum effort to solve the problem. Obviously there would need to be allowances made for extraordinary cases—a person who falls from a scaffold and breaks his back will need a longer time for treatment than will a person who sprained her ankle. The money saved by such a new system would put millions of dollars back into the compensation program to be used for people with truly serious disabling conditions.

Under the present system, if a patient is off the job more than six months, the possibility of returning to work decreases considerably. After a year, that person is unlikely to get back to work, no matter what you do. The important principle in Worker's Compensation cases is for the patient to be diagnosed and treated *early*, and to be returned to work before he or she becomes discouraged and the incentive to work disappears. When treatment drags out, it is a disaster for the patient and the family, and is of no benefit to the employer.

How Your Doctor Can Help Save Your Job

It is usually harder to find a new job than it is to keep the old one; therefore, have your doctor help keep your employer on your side so that your job will be waiting for you when your back is healed. For example, ask your doctor to let your employer know immediately what your diagnosis is (the doctor must have your permission to do this). And tell your doctor to keep your employer informed about your progress so your employer understands that you are truly taking steps toward recovery.

If your condition will take quite a while to heal, have your physician explain that you will probably have to take some time off for a period, but that afterward you are likely to be able to do the same job as well as you did before.

If your employer is not willing to keep you on and you belong to a union, have your doctor get in touch with your union.

If it turns out you won't be able to return to your old job because you have a permanent disability and can't handle your old job, you can have your doctor suggest to your employer that you can continue working and that you can be trained for some other type of work in the company.

Don't lose motivation and then start exaggerating your injury to gain more money or to keep from going back to a job. (Physicians sometimes say that the fastest way to get a patient well is to have his or her compensation settlement paid. They call it the "greenback poultice".)

It is natural to have what is called posttraumatic neurosis, a common reaction to serious physical injury. Days or weeks after the accident, the person suddenly realizes fully the threat to life and limb, and the peril he or she has been through, and it frequently causes a major personality upheaval. The person becomes anxious and irritable or outraged by the invasion of body and life by hidden perils. Police say that the same type of reaction occurs in people who have been assaulted or whose homes have been broken into, exposing them and their family to danger. Understanding that the reaction is common makes it easier for the victim and family to deal with it. Also, this will only be a temporary problem. You can avoid panic, knowing it will go away and you will be able to get back to normal again.

Remind your doctor frequently that you do not want to fall unnecessarily into a dependent role, that you want to get back to as full a function as possible in both your job and your family, and that you want to be independent and productive.

Glossary of Terms

A

Acetabulum   The socket of the pelvic bone.

ACTH   Adrenocorticotropic hormone, a secretion of the pituitary gland that stimulates the adrenal glands to greater activity. This causes an increase of the adrenal cortex hormones, including cortisone.

Acupressure   Japanese system of healing that involves finger pressure applied on several points on the acupuncture meridians of the body.

Acupuncture   A traditional method of Chinese medicine in which fine needles are inserted into the body in key points to release internal blockages and balance energy.

Acute   Term applied to short, severe attacks of a disease or of pain.

Adhesion   A fibrous band that connects two surfaces together that are normally separate.

Adjustment   A chiropractic manipulation to align the vertebrae of the spinal column properly.

Adrenal Glands   Endocrine glands that rest on the top of each kidney.

Adrenalin   A trade name for the substance secreted by the adrenal gland. This hormone becomes more plentiful in reactions of fear, rage, flight, or fight. Also called *epinephrine*.

-algia Painful.

Alternative Therapies Also called nontraditional therapies. Usually offered by a holistic practitioner of health care. The new more accurate term is complementary therapies; that is, patients and physicians should not consider them as alternates, but should use them as appropriate *with* other medical treatments.

Ambulatory Care Health services provided on an outpatient basis, in contrast to services provided to hospitalized patients (inpatients).

Analgesic Pain-relieving drug. The two most frequently used are aspirin and acetaminophen.

Anesthesiologist A physician who is specifically trained in the use of anesthetics.

Anesthetist A nonphysician who is trained in the use of anesthetics.

Ankylosing Spondylitis An inflammatory disease of the spine that has many of the characteristics of rheumatoid arthritis.

Ankylosis Consolidation and abnormal immobility of a joint.

Annulus Fibrosus The tough outermost part of the discs between the vertebrae and surrounding the nucleus pulposus in its center.

Anomaly An anatomical structure that is not normal.

Anterior Toward the front.

Anti-Inflammatory Any drug or other agent meant to decrease inflammation.

Arthralgia Pain in the joints without inflammation.

Arthritis Inflammation of a joint. Can be degenerative joint disease, osteathritis, gouty arthritis, rheumatoid arthritis, allergenic arthritis, and so on.

Arthro- A combining form denoting some relationship to a joint, where two bones meet.

Arthrodesis The fusion of a joint, an operative procedure sometimes applied to the spine to relieve pain and counteract instability.

Arthropathy Any joint disease.

Arthroscopy Surgical examination of the interior of a joint with an arthroscope, a small fiber-optic tube.

Asymmetry   Dissimilarity between two corresponding parts of the body.

Asymptomatic   Absence of symptoms.

Atlas   The first cervical (neck) vertebra; its major function is to support the skull.

Atrophy   Wasting away, as may be seen with lack of use of a part of the body.

Avascular   Absence of adequate blood supply.

Axis   The second cervical vertebra.

B

Benign   Term used to describe a growth that is harmless to surrounding tissue.

Biopsy   Removing a piece of tissue for microscopic inspection.

Body of Vertebra   The large block-shaped part of a vertebra.

C

Calcium Deposit   Place where crystals containing calcium occur as a response to inflammation or injury.

Cartilage   A form of connective tissue that is firm, but not hard and strong like bone. It usually covers the end of a joint and acts as a cushion. Gristle.

CAT, or CT, Scan   Computerized axial tomography that is 100 times more sensitive than an ordinary X ray and takes a cross-section view of the body.

Cauda Equina   The lower end of the spinal cord as it fans out to form the fifth lumbar nerve, the sacral nerves, and the coccygeal nerves. *Cauda equina* means "horse's tail" in Latin.

Cauda Equina Syndrome   Pressure on the nerves in the low back to produce multiple nerve root irritation and loss of bowel and bladder control. Requires immediate attention.

Cerebrospinal Fluid   Watery fluid that bathes brain and spinal cord; contained by the meninges.

Cervical   Referring to the neck.

Cervical Ribs   Extra ribs sometimes abnormally present in the neck area.

Cervical Spine Seven spinal segments between the base of the skull and the thoracic spine.

Chemonucleolysis The use of injected chemicals to dissolve portions of the intravertebral discs.

Chiropractic Treatment discipline based on the theory that many symptoms and disorders may be explained by spinal malalignment.

Chondral Plate Bone along the top and bottom surfaces of the body of each vertebra. Also called *end plate*.

Chondritis Inflammation of cartilage.

Chondro- A combining form denoting a relationship to cartilage.

Chronic A long-lasting condition.

Chronic Muscular Tension A long-term condition in which the muscle fibers are persistently held in a shortened, contracted state.

Chymopapain An enzyme derived from the papaya fruit, commonly used in the technique of chemonucleolysis.

Coccygodynia Pain in the region of the tailbone or coccyx.

Coccyx Three or four somewhat fixed fused segments at the end of the spine. The tailbone.

Collagen A protein formed in the body. Major component of scars, ligaments, tendons, and a portion of the bone.

Compression Crumbling or smashing of bone by forces acting parallel to the long axis of the bone; especially vertebral fractures.

Compression of the Nerve Root Pinching of nerve resulting from a tumor, fracture, or bulging disc. Pain from this type of disorder is called radicular pain.

Congenital Term applied to a condition present at birth.

Connective Tissues Tissues present throughout the body that act to bind one body part to another and fill the spaces between body parts.

Contrast Material Chemical used to fill spaces so they will show clearly on X rays. Sometimes called *dye*.

Cordotomy Incision into the nerve fiber tract within the spinal cord for relief of pain.

Cortex The hard outer shell of a bone.

Corticosteroid Anti-inflammatory drug, such as cortisone, used for short periods to reduce inflammation of the joints. These drugs are produced from a substance found in the adrenal glands.

Crick Sudden catch in the neck that produces inability or reluctance to rotate or tilt the head in certain directions.

D

Decompression Procedure to relieve pressure on the spinal cord or nerve roots.

Degenerative Tissue destruction as cell metabolism becomes overburdened with wastes and unable to take in new nutrients; usually associated with a deficiency in circulation to that area and a loss of function.

Diathermy Electromagnetic waves used as a means of producing heat deep inside tissues.

Disc Intervertebral disc. The joints between the vertebral bodies. Composed of a ring of ligaments (annulus fibrosus) and a center of semisolid gel (nucleus pulposus). Sometimes spelled "disk."

Disc Degeneration Changes in the invertebral disc resulting in loss of volume and water content of the nucleus pulposus. Often accompanied by narrowing of the space that the disc occupies between vertebral bodies.

Discectomy Operation to remove disc material.

Discogram X ray made with injection of opaque material into a disc between two vertebrae.

Dislocation Displacement of bones meeting at a joint. Bones are restored to their normal position by manipulation.

Dynamometer Test An instrument used to measure the strength of muscle contraction; such as the strength in the hand grip.

Dysfunction Absence of a normal function. Abnormal or irregular action.

E

Effusion Swelling within a joint caused by a fluid such as blood escaping into the body cavity.

Elasticity Property of being able to increase in length under stress and then return to the original length at rest.

Electromyograph (EMG) A record of muscle activity based on a measurement of its electrical responses.

End Plate The bone along the top and bottom surfaces of the body of each vertebra. Also called *chondral plate*.

Epidural Space The space inside the spinal column.

Epinephrine Adrenalin.

Erector Spinae Muscles The large muscles that run along the full length of the spine. These are the strongest of the back muscles and the most important for holding the back erect.

Ergonomics Study of body movement applied to the design of facilities, equipment, tools, and tasks for both efficiency and safety.

Etiology The cause of a disease.

Exacerbation Return to previous symptoms.

Extension Arching the trunk or neck backward or moving a joint to make the angle formed by its parts approach a straight line.

F

Facet Bony process on each side of the back of each vertebra.

Facet Joint Sites where the vertebrae join together at the back of the spine.

Fibro- Latin combining form indicating the presence of or association with fibrous tissue such as tendons and ligaments.

Fibromyositis A term sometimes used to describe a syndrome that among other symptoms includes muscular fatigue, soreness, and tender areas.

Fibrosis Condition of having an increase in the number of fibers and fiber cells in a tissue.

Fibrous Composed of fibers. Ropelike.

Flaccid Lack of tone.

Flexion Bending the trunk or neck forward or moving a joint to make the angle formed by its part smaller.

Flexor Muscle Muscle that bends a joint.

Fluoroscope An instrument for observing the internal body organs at work. X rays are passed through the body onto a screen where the shadows of organs can be seen and studied.

Foramen (pl. Forimina) Hole or window, usually through or between bones.

Foraminotomy An operation to enlarge a foramen.

Fusion An operation done to eliminate motion where it was previously present, usually by joining two vertebrae together.

G

Glioma Tumor arising from specialized connective tissue found in brain and spinal cord.

Gout A disease that affects the joints and kidneys, caused by an excess amount of uric acid in the body.

H

Hamstring Muscle Large muscles at the back of the thigh attached to the hip above and the leg below.

Hypertrophic Arthritis Ridging and spurring of bone near joints as evidence of wear and tear of these areas.

I

Iatrogenic Disorder Abnormal condition produced in a patient by the physican or medical, surgical, or pharmaceutical measures used.

Idiopathic Without a known cause.

Iliopsoas A composite of two muscles going from the back and hip to the thigh.

Indomethacin An anti-inflammatory drug.

Inflammation Reaction of the body or a part of the body to some kind of irritation. Characterized by swelling, increased temperature in the area, redness, and tenderness.

Intervertebral Disc The spongy fibrous cushions that join adjacent vertebral bodies and give spring to the spine.

Intervertebral Foramen Hole between sides of each vertebra through which spinal nerves pass.

Ischemia Insufficient blood supply to a tissue or organ.

Isometric Without movement. Usually referring to exercises done by creating tension against resistance, without movement.

J

Joint Mice Loose pieces of cartilage or other organic material in a joint.

K

Kummell's Disease Progressive wedging of the body of a vertebra after injury. This disease usually represents an unrecognized or untreated fracture.

Kyphosis Curvature of the spine. Humpback.

L

Lamina Portion of the vertebra that makes up the roof over the vertebral canal.

Laminectomy An operation to remove the back roof or lamina portion of a vertebra. Technically "laminectomy" means removal of the entire lamina structure of the vertebra, but the term most often is used to refer to any operation that approaches the vertebral canal from the back.

Laminotomy Formation of a hole in the lamina without disruption of the continuity of the entire lamina in order to approach the intervertebral disc.

Lateral To the side or from the side.

Lesion Tissue or part of an organ damaged by injury or disease, usually with partial loss of function, for example, a bruise or broken bone.

Ligaments Sheets and strands of dense fibers that keep the joint ends together, completely enclosing the joint in a capsulelike arrangement.

Ligamentum Flavum Ligament that connects one vertebra to the next, forming part of the "roof" of the back of the spine. Also called "yellow ligament."

List Leaning to one side or another when standing or walking; commonly seen in lumbar disc disease.

Locked Back Syndrome Episodes of sudden, painful fixation of the lower back, which can be caused by a variety of mechanical problems.

Lordosis Backward curvature of the lumbar spine.

Lumbago An obsolete term meaning back pain.

Lumbar Puncture A testing and treatment procedure. A needle is used to measure the pressure of the cerebrospinal fluid, withdraw some of the fluid for examination, or introduce medications or anesthetic into the space surrounding the spinal cord in the low back region.

Lumbar Spine Five vertebra in the lower back. They provide most of the bending and turning ability of the back and bear most of the weight of the body.

Lumbosacral Joint The connection between the last lumbar and the first sacral vertebra.

Luxation Dislocation of bone or bones at joint site.

M

Magnetic Resonance Imaging (MRI) MRI is a diagnostic technology that uses a superconducting magnet and a computer to precisely image internal soft body tissue.

Malignant A tumor that is destructive and tends to spread throughout the body.

Manipulation A twisting or stretching action to attempt a favorable change in the position or movement of muscles, joints, or bones.

Marie-Strumpell Disease Inflammation of the spine, occurring as a rheumatoid-type disease in children.

Masseur A man who practices massage.

Masseuse A woman who practices massage.

Medial Toward the midline of the body.

Meninges The three layers of tissue that cover the brain and spinal cord and form the meningeal sac.

Meningitis Inflammation of the covering of the brain and spinal cord resulting from infectious agents such as bacteria, fungi, or viruses.

Mixed Arthritis When rheumatoid arthritis and osteoarthritis occur at the same time. This is usually caused by rheumatoid arthritis leading to osteoarthritis due to injury to the joints.

Morbidity Degree of illness; the ratio of sick to well persons.

Mortality Death rate.

Motor Points Areas where nerves join muscles. May coincide with trigger points and acupressure points.

Multiple Myeloma Multiple plasma cell tumors in bone, usually malignant.

Muscle Atrophy A general loss of muscle from various causes; muscle wasting.

Muscle Guarding Involuntary contraction of muscle in effort to avoid pain that would be produced by moving the body part.

Muscle Relaxants Group of drugs used to relieve pain caused by muscle tension.

Muscle Spasm Sudden contraction of muscle, usually in reflex response to stimulus from external source, for example, back spasm caused by a bulging disc.

Myalgia Pain in the muscles.

Myelography The injection of radio-opaque medium into the vertebral canal, to show disc protrusions or tumors that would not otherwise be seen on X rays.

Myodynia Pain in the muscles; myalgia; myosalgia.

Myopathy Any disease of muscles.

Myospasm Muscle spasm.

N

Necrosis Death of a tissue.

Neoplasm Abnormal new growth of tissue, either benign or malignant. A tumor.

Nerve Conduction Test Electrical test to determine the speed that an electrical impulse travels along a nerve.

Neural Arch The bony ring extending back from each vertebra, surrounding and protecting part of the spinal cord or the spinal nerves.

Neuralgia Severe pain along the course of a nerve not associated with any obvious or demonstrable structural changes in the nerve.

Neuritis Inflammation of a nerve, usually painful.

Neuro- Pertaining to the body's nervous system.

Neurogenic Originating in the nervous system.

Neurologist   Medical doctor who specializes in diagnoses and medical treatment of disorders involving the brain, spinal cord, and nerves.

Neuroma   Benign tumor of a nerve.

Neuropathy   Any disease of the nerves.

Neurosurgeon   Surgeon who specializes in diagnosis and care, including surgical operations, of disorders of the brain, spinal cord, and nerves.

Nerve Roots   Nerves that join the spinal cord and course through the vertebral canal. Anterior and posterior roots at each level join to form a "spinal nerve."

Neuroma   A benign tumor of a nerve.

Nonsteroidal Anti-Inflammatory Drugs (NSAIDs)   Drugs used against inflammation, such as in arthritis.

Nucleus Pulposus   The semiliquid gelatinous center of an intervertebral disc. Its major function is to provide a cushion between the vertebrae.

O

Orthopedic   Anything related to the correction of a deformity or disorder of the spine, arms, and legs.

Orthopedics   The medical specialty that deals with the treatment and prevention of disorders of the musculoskeletal system, which includes bones, muscles, joints, ligaments, tendons, and related structures.

Orthopedic Surgeon   Surgeon who specializes in diagnosis and care, including surgical operations, of deformities and disorders of the arms, legs, and spine.

Orthotics   Devices to straighten or balance the foot.

Osteoalgia   Pain within a bone.

Osteitis   Inflammation of bone with enlargement, tenderness, dull aching; there are many varieties.

Osteoarthritis   A disease of the joints that involves a breakdown of cartilage and other tissues. Inflammation may or may not be present.

Osteoarthropathy   A condition of increased bone formation at the joints; sometimes used to refer to osteoarthritis.

Osteochondritis Inflammation of both bone and cartilage.

Osteogenesis Imperfecta Condition in which bones are abnormally brittle and subject to fractures.

Osteomalacia An abnormal softening of the bone caused by lack of the bone-strengthening materials calcium and phosphorus. Generally caused by a deficiency in vitamin D.

Osteomyelitis Inflammation of bone marrow, cortex, tissue, and periosteum; can be caused by bacteria or fungus.

Osteonecrosis Death of bone tissue.

Osteopathy Medical discipline that teaches spinal manipulation as a treatment for many disorders, as well as medicines and surgery. The practitioner has a D.O. (doctor of osteopathy) rather than an M.D. (doctor of medicine) degree.

Osteoporosis Abnormal rarefaction of bone resulting from the failure of osteoblasts to lay down bone matrix; caused by age, disuse, trauma, or other disease.

Osteopetrosis An inherited disease characterized by a generalized increase in bone density that begins during growth. There are at least two different forms, one of early onset with poor prognosis, the other of late onset, little disability, and normal life expectancy.

Osteophyte Enlargement of a bone at its edge where ligaments attach. Sometimes called a "bone spur."

P

Paget's Disease (Osteitis Deformans) A disease associated with painful enlargement and deformity of the bones, often affecting the lumbar spine.

Paraplegia Paralysis of lower part of body or lower extremities.

Parathesia Abnormal sensation of numbness, prickling, burning, crawling, or tickling.

Passive Exercise Exercise done wholly by the use of outside force without using your own muscles to participate in the exercise.

Pedicle Side-wall portion of vertebra. Each vertebra has a right and left pedicle joining the body to the laminae and facets.

Pelvic Bones Bones that join to form the pelvis. The pelvis is formed from three bones grown together on each side—the ilium, ischium, and pubis.

Pelvic Tilt Rolling the pelvis forward and upward by flattening the lower back, pulling in and tightening the abdomen, and squeezing the buttocks together.

Physiatrist A physician who specializes in physical medicine; often develops a program of exercises for arthritic or other patients to help prevent crippling.

Physical Therapist A person trained to treat patients by physical means, such as heat, massage, exercise, whirlpool baths.

Pinprick Test Checks ability to feel a pinprick and the ability to determine the difference between sharp and dull.

Placebo Inert substance sometimes given to a study group of patients as part of a drug study. Patients are said to exhibit the "placebo effect" when their health status improves despite the fact the substance they are taking is inert.

Polo Belt A broad-backed belt designed to protect and support the low back area.

Polyneuritis Inflammation of multiple nerves.

Posterior Toward the back.

Prednisone A powerful corticosteroid sometimes used in the treatment of arthritis. It must be used under a doctor's direction to prevent serious side effects.

Prevalence The number of cases of a given disease existing in a given population at a specified moment of time.

Primary Osteoarthritis Osteoarthritis that occurs without having been influenced by any known event or injury; starts by itself.

Procaine The same as Novocain, a local anesthetic.

Processes When referring to bone, indicates outgrowths on the bones that serve as attachments for tendons and ligaments.

Pronate To turn inward.

Pronation Ankles roll inward, causing extra pressure on many of the muscles and bones of the feet, legs, and knees.

Prone Lying face down.

Prosthesis An artificial substitute for a body part, such as a leg, tooth, heart valve, or blood vessel. The plural form is prostheses.

Psychosomatic Pertaining to the influence of the mind and emotions upon the functions of the body, especially in relation to disease.

Q

Quadratus Lumborum The four-sided muscle that forms a flat sheet on each side of the spinal column and goes from the lower border to the last rib to the crest of the hipbone.

R

Radiculitis Inflammation of the origin of a nerve.

Radiculopathy Disease at the origin of a nerve, for example, by pain caused by a bulging disc in the spine.

Radioisotope A radioactive form of an element.

Radioisotopic Scanning Diagnostic technique involving radioactive labeling of tissues and organs by the injection of radioisotopes into the bloodstream. The emitted radioactivity is detected by a scanner and a record or "scan" of the labeled area is made.

Range of Motion (ROM) Exercises Designed to maintain or increase the amount of movement in a joint.

Recommended Daily Allowances (RDAs) The minimum daily requirements of vitamins and minerals as developed approximately every five years by the Food and Nutrition Board of the National Academy of Sciences. They are the minimum daily amounts needed to prevent disease, based on a 150-pound male adult engaged in light physical activity.

Referred Pain Pain felt some distance away from its cause. For example, pain in the knees caused by an arthritic hip.

Rehabilitation The return of a person disabled by accident or disease to physical, mental, emotional, social, and economic usefulness, and, if employable, to an opportunity for gainful employment.

Reiter's Syndrome A disease involving inflammation of the urethra and eyelids, plus arthritis.

Remission State when a disease appears to have gone away by itself, often temporarily.

Rheumatism Unspecific or unexplained aches and pains that may occur in joints and muscles or both; often used to mean arthritis.

Rheumatoid Arthritis Inflammation of the joints in which the whole body can be affected. Symptoms include stiffness and aching of joints, general fatigue, and loss of appetite.

Rheumatologist A physician who specializes in the treatment and management of patients with arthritis.

Rhizotomy Division of the roots of the spinal nerves.

Rhomboids Muscles from the back to the shoulder blades.

Rotator Cuff Cuff of tendons from the shoulder blade to the upper arm that control shoulder motion.

Rupture A breaking out from the normal confines.

S

Sacral Having to do with the sacrum.

Sacral Spine The five fused segments of the lower spine that connect to the pelvis.

Sacroiliac The joints or articulations between the sacrum and the two ilia of the pelvis, bound together by ligaments.

Sacrum The wedge-shaped bone at the back of the pelvis supporting the lumbar spine and ending in the coccyx (tailbone).

Scapula The shoulder blade.

Schuermann's Disease Inflammation of the cartilage of the lower thoracic and upper lumbar spine, causing pain.

Sciatica Pain along the sciatic nerve or part of it; may be in the buttocks, leg, or toes. Radiculopathy.

Scoliosis A sideways (lateral) curvature of the spine.

Secondary Osteoarthritis Osteoarthrisis that occurs because of wear and tear or injury to one or more joints.

Segment A portion or section of anything. In the spine, it refers to two adjoining vertebrae.

Shiatsu A Japanese form of acupressure that uses various finger pressure massage techniques on points along the meridians.

Sign Any objective evidence of a disease.

Slipped Disc A common name for bulging of part of the cushion disc between the vertebrae.

Soft, or Low-Impact, Aerobics Exercise without jolting up-and-down movements.

Spasm Muscle tightness that is not under voluntary control.

Spastic Characterized by spasms or tightening of the muscles.

Glossary

Spina Bifida A congenital failure of the vertebral bone to form completely. In severe cases this may allow the nerve tissues to protrude through the spine.

Spinal Column The backbone, composed of vertebrae; it protects the spinal cord.

Spinal Cord The main trunk line for nerve messages to and from the brain, extending through, and protected by, the vertebrae of the backbone.

Spinal Disc The fibrous connective tissue with a gel-like interior located between each vertebrae that acts like a shock absorber for the spine.

Spinal Nerves Nerves running from the spinal cord to various parts of the body. There are 31 pairs of spinal nerves.

Spinal Stenosis Abnormal narrowing of the spinal canal so that the nerves that normally pass through do not have adequate space.

Spine The bony structure of the back including the ligaments that bind together the 33 vertebral bones of which it is composed.

Spinous Process Posteriormost bone projection of the spine. It is the part of the spine that can be felt through the skin.

Splint A rigid structure applied to a part of the body to immobilize that area.

Spondylarthritis Arthritis of the spine.

Spondylitis Inflammation of the spine. May refer either to infection or inflammation from other causes such as arthritis.

Spondylosis Condition of the spine characterized by osteophytes, bone thickening, and disc degeneration.

Spondylolisthesis An unhealed fracture across the back of a vertebra, usually the last lumbar, which makes this part of the back unstable. It is usually congenital, but may be caused by an injury.

Spondylotic Myelopathy Impairment of spinal cord function because of narrowing of the vertebral canal as a result of spondylosis.

Sprain A wrenching of a joint that tears or severely stretches the ligaments with bleeding and swelling.

Spur Rough edge on bone, or ligament that has turned to bone at the site of its attachments to bone. Also called *osteophyte*.

Standing Pelvic Tilt Flattening of the lower back, pulling in of the abdomen, and rolling forward and upward with the pelvis, while standing.

Stenosis   A narrowing of an opening.

Steroid   A group of chemicals, including cortisone, that has chemical structures and physiological effects similar to hormones produced by the adrenal cortex.

Steroidal   Having the structure and properties of steroids.

Strain   Overstretching of muscle fibers caused by overexercising or overexerting some part of the musculature.

Stress   Physical, chemical, or emotional factors that may cause bodily or mental tension; also, gradual fracture caused by repeated or prolonged stress.

Subluxation   Partial dislocation of bones at a joint. The bones return to their normal position without assistance; also, chronic persistence of the tendency of a bone to become dislocated.

Supination   Ankles roll toward the outside of the body, causing extra pressures for the feet, legs, and knees.

Supine   Face up. Lying on the back.

Symptom   Any subjective evidence of a patient's condition.

Syndrome   A set of symptoms that occur together and are therefore given a name to indicate that particular combination.

Synovial Fluid   The colorless lubricating fluid contained in a joint or a bursa. When the body pumps out too much synovial fluid during an injury, there is swelling. "Water on the knee."

Synovitis   Inflammation of the synovial membrane.

T

Tendon   A fibrous cord of connective tissue that attaches muscles to bone.

Tendinitis   Inflammation of tendons.

Thoracic   Pertaining to the chest.

Thoracic Vertebrae   The 12 spinal vertebrae in the upper back corresponding to the 12 ribs of the thorax.

Thorax   The chest.

Torticollis   A contracted state of the cervical muscles producing tension of the neck. Wryneck.

Tomography Technique to show detailed images of structures lying in a predetermined plane of tissue, while eliminating detail of images of structures in other planes.

Traction A pulling, stretching force usually used in attempt to stretch tight muscles, ligaments, or joints.

Transverse Process Bony projection of the vertebrae for muscle attachment.

Trauma Wound or injury.

Trigger Spot An area of tenderness in the muscle that produces pain when pressure is applied to it.

Trunk The body except for arms, legs, and head. Torso.

U

Ultrasonography Medical use of sound waves to display structures within the body. The technique is often used to determine fetal age or to detect abnormalities of structures.

Ultrasound High-frequency sound vibrations, not audible to the human ear.

Uric Acid A chemical compound that is a product of metabolism in the body; an excess of this acid can form crystallized deposits in the joints and tissues, as in gout.

V

Vascular Pertaining to the blood vessels.

Vertebrae The bones of the spine.

Vertebral Body The main portion of vertebrae.

Vertebral Canal Tunnel through the spine from the head to the tailbone. Through it pass the spinal cord and spinal nerves.

W

Wryneck Tilting and rotation of the head. Torticollis.

Y

Yellow Ligament Ligament that connects one lamina to the next, thus forming part of the back roof of the spine. Has a yellow color and unusual amount of elasticity. Also called *ligamentum flavum*.

Yoga A philosophic and treatment-oriented system based on the interconnection of body, mind, and spirit. It involves a system focusing on postures, stretches, cleansing techniques, breathing, and a mental/spiritual system focusing on concentration and letting go of unnecessary emotion.

Index

Index

Index

Index